12/17/14

FOR Maggie,
and Paul

The Bend in the Road

Lenny Burke's Farm

Love, Emmie & Love, Lenny
+ even more love,
Yvonne Daley

The Bend in the Road

The Story of Lenny Burke's Farm

ISBN: 978-1-60571-234-5

Cover Photo: © 2014 Tai Lam
Back Cover Photo: © 2014 Christian Wideawake
Design: Debbi Wraga
Copy Editor: Andrea Rundgren

Photo of Lenny Burke with James Brady, printed by permission to H.I.S. from John Spragens Jr.
Photo of Vanessa Doggett, page 108, Cassandra Hotaling Hahn, Rutland Herald.
All other photos: Yvonne Daley, Sue Sharp, Jessica Franzoni, Kathy Chandler, Lenny Burke's Farm.

Graphs and information on pages 59, 85, 97, and 103 are reproduced with permission from the US Centers for Disease Control and Prevention and The Brain Injury Foundation. Information on Page 84 is reprinted with permission from the Delaware Health and Social Services of the Division of Services for Aging and Adults with Physical Disabilities. Rancho Los Amigos created the Levels of Cognitive Functioning guide found on page 80.

Proceeds from this book will benefit Lenny Burke's Farm, Wallingford, Vermont, and its satellite programs.

Also by Yvonne Daley

An Independent Man, with Sen. James M. Jeffords
Vermont Writers: A State of Mind
Octavia Boulevard
A Mighty Storm

Note to readers: A narrative that tells Lenny Burke's story runs throughout the book. Sidebars (with lavender border) provide snapshots of clients and staff and provide educational information about brain injuries.

Available at Northshire Bookstore • www.northshire.com

Printed in the United States of America

Early praise for *The Bend in the Road*

Yvonne Daley's *Octavia Boulevard*, a memoir, was an *artistic* triumph that read like Dickens in San Francisco. *The Bend in the Road* is a *journalistic* triumph, an extremely important, deeply humanistic statement in these otherwise rather dark, silly, solipsistic, and cynical times. The two books share an unself-centeredness almost unheard of in this era. *The Bend in the Road* is the remarkable story of Lenny Burke and his courageous battle to recover from a brain injury suffered during a high-school basketball game. Along the way, Daley – a prize-winning journalist and author – introduces us to other residents of Lenny Burke's Farm, a renowned rehabilitative center combining state-of-the-art treatment with love and respect for human dignity, to do what often seems downright impossible. It's a beautifully written celebration of hope and joy in the face of just about the worst life can do to us.

—Howard Frank Mosher, author of ten novels, including three adapted into movies, *Disappearances, A Stranger in the Kingdom* and *Where the Rivers Run North.*

The Bend In The Road is not about the tragedy that befalls an adolescent, Lenny Burke, at the prime of his life, but rather about the "rebirth" of an individual and the life-changing forces that many others experience right alongside him. Lenny's story is gut wrenching, poignant, motivating, and captivating. It is the story of what individuals, families, and entire communities can do to "move mountains" when necessary and when their hearts are in it. As people say, "bad things roll down hill," but so do good things. Lenny Burke is one of those good things that changed the world around him for the better. Lenny's story will bend your heart and soul.

—Dr. Ron Savage, president, Sarah Jane Brain Foundation; chair, International Pediatric Brain Injury Society; board of governors, International Brain Injury Association.

The Bend In The Road offers a bird's eye view of love in daily action on many levels. We are drawn into the story of Emmie's love for her oldest son Lenny and the Burke family, friends and associates whose 'yes' served his healing process and later Lenny Burke's Farm and Emma's Place. In true practical Vermont fashion, each and all got to work. In the process, they innovated and then documented what they learned, tried and what worked—thus beginning what has turned into a number of movements to serve the brain-injured. *The Bend in the Road* not only tells Lenny's, Emmie's and others' moving stories, it educates us as to how widespread brain injuries are – hundreds of thousands annually; it reminds us of the great need to prevent brain injuries; how important it is to continue to do research on treatment and rehabilitation; and as we saw with Emmie's vision—how very important it is to have rehabilitation centers that feel just like home because they are home.

—Cecile G. Betit ,Ph.D., researcher, forthcoming book *Making Change in the Real World: Carris Reels Transition to a 100% Employee Owned and Governed Company.*

Yvonne Daley has gifted us a thorough and thoughtful account of Lenny Burke's remarkable and brave journey, the complicated challenges met by his loving family, the resulting crusade championed by his courageous and compassionate mother, and the warm embrace of a loving community. Yvonne's gripping story will allow you to feel like you are part of this amazing extended family, led by Emmie Burke and her children and colleagues. They transformed a community, and they rocked the world of brain injury research and action, by turning what was a life threatening injury into a life of meaning and purpose for Lenny and all of us whose lives have been enriched by their loving example.

—David Wolk, president, *Castleton State College.*

The Lenny Burke's Farm purpose statement written by the clients and recited at weekly group meetings:

Recovery: Lenny Burke's Farm.
There is no place like home. We are all family.
A circle of friends.
Everybody knows your name.
Everyone in the circle respects each other.
A circle of faith, love, harmony, hope and joy.
Recovery: Nobody wins alone.
Courage does not always roar.
Sometimes it is a quiet voice at the end of the day,
saying, "I will try again tomorrow."
We all have hope for a better tomorrow.

The Bend in the Road

Lenny Burke's Farm

Yvonne Daley

Verdant
Rutland, Vermont & San Francisco

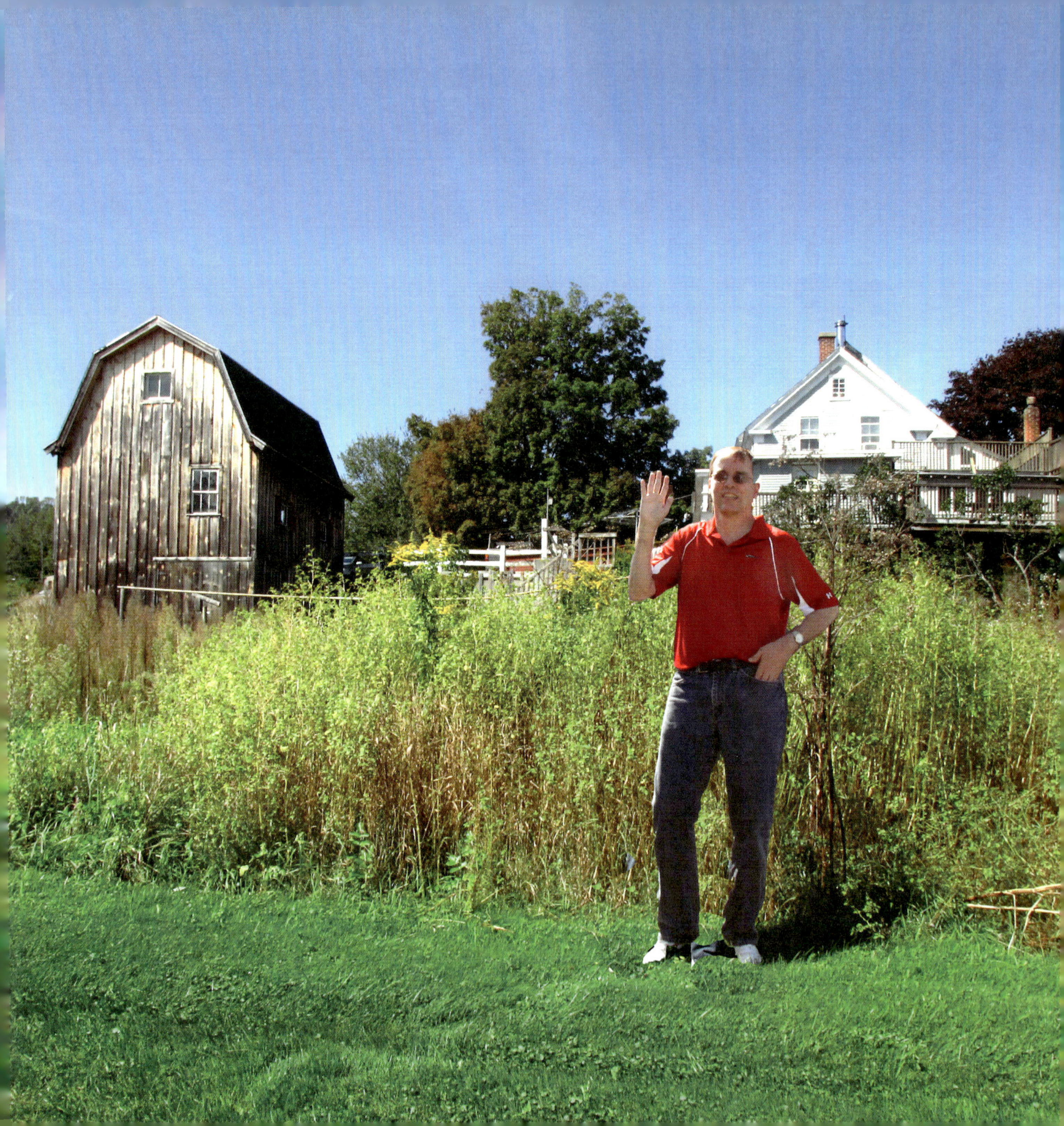

Prologue

Emmie Burke and her children, Lenny, Kevin, Michael and Kathy, and I started talking about a book about Lenny Burke and Lenny Burke's Farm years ago, the idea being that this story of one almost unimaginable trauma and a family's response is the kind of story we need now, perhaps more than ever, a story of unselfishness and perseverance, a singular story that has brought healing, real healing, directly to hundreds and, indirectly, to countless others.

Nearly everyone who was living in our part of Vermont in 1979 has heard the story of the promising young man undercut by an opponent in a high school basketball game, the resulting coma as he lay near death, the seemingly miraculous recovery. Others closer to the event had followed the parents' and siblings' anguish, the dedication of friends and teachers who lived for weeks outside the intensive care unit, hanging on every piece of information. Still others knew of a mother's creativity and inventiveness, using smelly sneakers and pizza to communicate with a son who only appeared silent to those who weren't listening with more than their ears, and then the journey to share what was learned with others.

Lenny Burke's injury, an injustice that might cause one to question not just his or her faith but the very meaning of what it is to be alive, was a pebble that weighed an immeasurable quantity; the pool it was propelled into is, also, immeasurable, the ripples of such significance that there's no way of knowing how many lives have been affected by what one child, one family and one community learned, not just about tenacity and inventiveness, but what scientists, therapists, mental health practitioners, parents and survivors have also learned about that remarkable part of our body we call the brain.

As I, too, entered the journey with the Burke family, following that bend in the road, it became clear that Lenny's injury, like the proverbial pebble in the pool, generated an ever-widening circle of questions about the brain: How is it that this organ that weighs roughly 3.3 pounds can do

"It's not what happens to us that makes a difference ... It's how we choose to respond to it that makes all the difference."

—The Rev. Richard Marceau

so much or, more precisely, how do those billions of neurons in our brain – roughly 86 billion! – communicate with one another and with the rest of the body? How, if the frontal lobes of the brain control most executive functions such as self-control, planning, reasoning and abstract thought, can people who have suffered disastrous damage to this area of the brain relearn these skills? What is going on in the brain when a person is in a coma and how much of what they recall from that time is real? And what of that phenomenon we call a near-death experience?

I have spent much of the past year hanging out at Lenny Burke's Farm, Emma's Place and its satellite residences created by the Burkes for the rehabilitation of others who sustained head injuries, pondering these questions in the company of people with a host of what are called disabilities. Some can't walk. Others have difficulty talking. Still others can't remember what they had for breakfast. Others, who themselves sustained traumatic injuries to their brains, are caring for people still in recovery.

I have no words to express what a joy it has been, what pleasure I've had watching Vanessa compose a pithy diatribe on her Dynavox or when Danny flashes the peace sign and graces me with his positive benediction; to hear Meredith talk about stem-cell research and Geep sing the 20 or so verses of "The Weight" while the aroma of whatever delicious dinner Linda has made fills the air. All the while, Christopher Patrick Russell – I love to say his full name because it always makes him smile – beams his beatific grin, hand raised and fingers spread in the Mork from Ork salute.

Just this summer, Buddy, a man whose brain was said to have almost died from lack of oxygen, began to speak more words and walk with more confidence; he's smiling a lot and seems less afraid. Some days he looks downright happy. Jason is chopping wood and finishing a carving of a cat and kittens with his wood-burning tool. Paul is selling tomatoes and zucchini he grew for spending money; Louise is riding the bus to bingo at the senior center; David has seen the tree planted over Lizzie's grave flower. Some of the clients have become grandparents; two are in love; one is moving closer to home.

Every book is a journey. You begin with an idea, an inclination to explore something interesting and important, to tell a story, a tale worth telling, and then set forth. I write nonfiction so, unlike my novelist friends, I talk a lot about what I'm working on, inviting friends and colleagues into the adventure, seeking their company and reflections on the odyssey. Over the decades, it's been universally true that these conversations will open up new ways of looking at my subject, lead me along an unexplored itinerary, reveal the oversights in my assumptions, and teach me new ways of understanding what I thought I'd fully explored.

Serendipity comes in many forms; you just have to keep a lookout for the ways in which it will enrich your work and, in so doing, your life. Nearly everyone I've spoken to about this book knows someone who has sustained a traumatic brain injury, or they have had one themselves. It's the way we live our lives: cars, sports, war, assault, stupidity, birth defects and aging blood vessels, simply being in the wrong place at the wrong time, or the right place at the right time.

So, yes, this is Lenny Burke's story, but also yours.

—*Yvonne Daley*

"Experience is not what happens to a man; it is what a man does with what happens to him."

—*Aldous Huxley*

Acknowledgments

It goes without saying that literally hundreds of people have contributed to this book since Lenny Burke's injury in 1979, from the Rutland, Vermont, residents who donated funds for his rehabilitation, and the friends, colleagues, parents, teachers, doctors, therapists and others, here in Vermont and across the country, whose support has been immeasurable over the decades. Our thanks also to the scientists and therapists throughout the country whose breakthroughs in the treatment of traumatic brain injury have helped so many. May their work be supported.

We owe a special debt of gratitude to Sue Sharp, who helped with so many tasks from scanning photos to gathering lost documents. Immense gratitude to Debbi Wraga, whose design and attention to detail are evident on every page. We also want to thank the town of Wallingford and its residents, who have over the decades treated our staff and clients with patience and dignity, embraced our presence in your community, and participated in the rehabilitation of people with traumatic brain injuries.

This book is dedicated to the memory of Rev. Richard Marceau and his wife Ellen Marceau, who taught us all about the power of serendipity and love; to the Wolk family – Doctor Arthur Wolk, Florrie Wolk and David Wolk – who walked the journey with us; to Dr. Peter Upton, who may not have been a believer but who never stopped trying to save Lenny's life; to Dr. Ron Savage, whose instincts in the care of TBI have helped literally thousands; to Bill Frey, a psychologist who discovered music's ability to help restore memory long before it was accepted practice; to Marion and John Austin, who know the meaning of friendship; to the therapists at the Vermont Achievement Center and Rancho Los Amigos, whose treatments made so much difference; to the clients whose presence has enriched Lenny's life and that of his family; to the parents and guardians who have trusted Lenny Burke's Farm with the care of their loved ones; and to the staff of Lenny Burke's Farm who show up day after day, cheerful, positive and professional, making a difference.

"We all thought after intensive rehabilitation that Lenny would return to Rutland "all better" and his life would go on as before. Yes, Lenny was out of coma, he was walking and talking, but he was not "all better." His life had permanently changed because of his traumatic brain injury."

—Ron Savage

The Bend in the Road

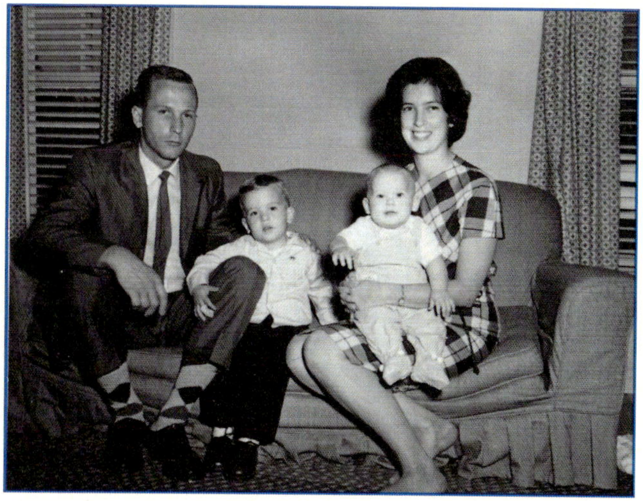

It was a wonderful family. Not perfect, of course, as nothing, alas, is, but Len and Emmie Burke considered themselves quite fortunate as they began their lives together in the small and close-knit town of Chittenden in the magical state of Vermont. Local sweethearts, the couple married in 1960 when Emmie was just 18 and Len 23. Young people both far and near were just beginning to bring big changes to the American culture, but Len and Emmie Burke were not children of the Sixties; they had been born just a little too early for the long hair and bell bottoms and, given their natures, were unlikely to step out of societal norms. Besides, with four children born in the first eight years of their marriage, the couple had little time for strobe-lit concerts or political demonstrations. For them, community, family and church were central elements of their lives. Nonetheless, the values of those times and the goals – peace, social justice, equality, community and harmony – informed their lives and work. They embraced the best parts of the social changes that were transforming America and in their own quiet way celebrated the fact that their children had been born into a world where people of all ethnicities and religions, both men and women, were demanding greater freedom and more equal opportunities.

Like most women of the time, Emmie was a stay-at-home mom, which was a wonderful thing as the couple's first son, Lenny John, or just plain Lenny as he will be called in this book – he was named after his father, who went by Len – was a little spitfire. From his earliest months, friends and family members often remarked how smart and happy Lenny was, so full of energy and strength. He was one of those kids who gave their parents something fresh to brag about each day and his father, who worked as a television repairman and carpenter, loved bringing stories of his son's newest conquests along on his house calls.

Lenny's coordination and physical strength were evident right away; he pulled himself up to a standing position in his wooden playpen at six months of age and walked by eight and a half months. But there was something more about young Lenny, something that set him apart from most youngsters. It wasn't just his intelligence, but more his sense of self and his role in the small universe of the family. This confidence was a natural attribute but it was strengthened by his mother's determination to teach him not just the usual lessons of childhood like the alphabet, numbers and colors, but more complex concepts and information. By the age of three, for example, Lenny could recite the Pledge of Allegiance with complete assurance, pronouncing each word carefully as if he understood its meaning. Indeed, there were few who heard his recitation who weren't convinced he did understand every word. When President Kennedy was assassinated, Lenny was the same age as John-John and watched the television with such serious intent that his parents thought he was following what was going on.

Lenny's ability to memorize and parse out meaning wasn't the only characteristic that set him aside, not just from other children but also from other people his parents knew, even those much, much older. Just as his mother was a bit obsessed with teaching Lenny what she knew, Lenny was passionate about sharing what he had been taught with his siblings, quite aware at the earliest age of his role as the big brother. While many first children are less than eager to share the limelight, Lenny was keen to shine the spotlight on his younger brother Kevin, born just 19 months after Lenny.

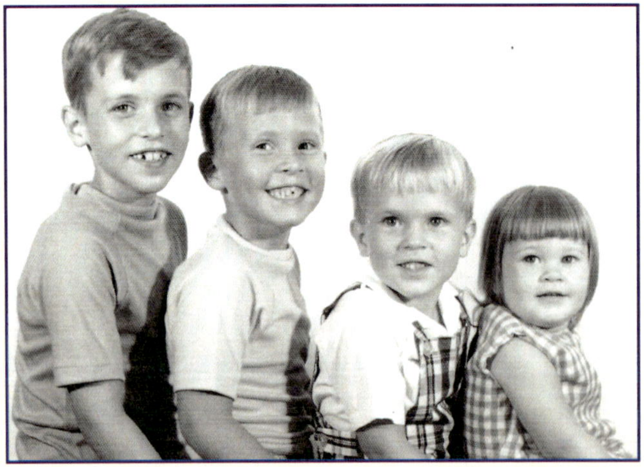

Lenny, Kevin, Michael and Kathleen Burke.

Emmie recalls the day during naptime when she heard Lenny and Kevin, then just 18 months old, chatting rather than sleeping. Stopping at the bedroom door before admonishing them, Emmie was astonished to hear Kevin repeat the whole Pledge of Allegiance. Lenny had taught it to him and was now coaching him on his delivery. Now there was a new story for Len to share with customers and friends. When the next baby, Michael, arrived, Lenny, now four years old, and Kevin, two and a half, were convinced that it was their job to pass on the knowledge. The family story goes that Kevin squeezed Michael's cheeks so much he still has dimples. Lenny had passed on his sense of sharing the attention to Kevin, who passed it on to Michael.

And then, into this house with three sons came Kathy, the Princess. Lenny adored her while her other two brothers pretended they were not quite convinced that having a girl in the house was such a great idea. Of course, Emmie and Len were thrilled to have a daughter to complete the family. Four kids in six and a half years might have seemed daunting, but the Burkes were surrounded by family members and a tight-knit community that seems almost storybook quality today.

To fully understand this story, you first need to imagine the community of Chittenden, Vermont, the largest town by area in all of Vermont, and then you've got to understand the city of Rutland, the county seat. Then as now, the smaller towns surrounding Rutland City maintained general and corner stores but most commerce took place in Rutland, a working class community with a handsome brick downtown where residents and shoppers knew the people they encountered each day. Rutland was also a sports town and its two high schools – the public Rutland High School and the private and Catholic Mount Saint Joseph Academy – were cross-city rivals with MSJ, as the smaller of the two, often playing the scrappy underdog.

The town of Chittenden had been named for Thomas Chittenden, one of the Green Mountain Boys who fought against Great Britain in the War of Independence and became Vermont's first governor. It is one of 28 towns surrounding Rutland City but, given its wide and rural terrain and the fact that the town is nearly split in two by a ridge of the Green Mountains, it evolved into a community of many semi-autonomous hamlets. Less than 1,000 people populated its nearly 75 square miles in the late 1960s; the population is roughly 1,200 now. Chittenden also has a beautiful manmade reservoir that's open to the public for recreation. Much of the town is wooded and the wilder parts on the eastern side – a rare tract of unbroken forest – have been incorporated into the Green Mountain National Forest.

For young children growing up here, the area was rich with deep woods and secret places to explore. Young families like the Burkes quickly formed small playgroups and learning circles; the children were like cousins to one another, going on from the local elementary school to attend either Rutland High or MSJ. There was lots of unorganized play as well and time for daredevil shenanigans. Emmie cringes when she hears the story of how the children would jump into the family's below-ground swimming pool from the garage roof or the time Kevin "rode" his horse Suzy Q across Chittenden Dam's deep waters, accompanied by his siblings swimming alongside, holding another horse.

Emmie had grown up and received her early training in juggling many roles as a young girl here. Her mother, Dorothy Ormsbee, had moved to Chittenden in the early 1950s when Emmie was just 11 and her sister, Hannah, two years younger. Dorothy had married quite late in life to a 63-year-old man with two sons from a previous marriage. Dorothy was 38 when Emmie was born, 40 when she gave birth to Hannah. It's hard to understand today why this situation was considered rather scandalous at the time, but it was. Dorothy was quite independent, however, and didn't let others' opinions bother her. When her husband died, she decided to leave Ticonderoga, NY, where his family lived, and move to the relative wilderness of Chittenden. Much as she enjoyed making her own decisions, she had little practical skills for managing the home and two young children on her own. Beyond that, she had to earn the family's income. She served as the Chittenden Town Clerk for many years while also working other jobs, including at the Brandon Training School, a former state facility for people with mental retardation. While Emmie dismisses her role as the little mother, her sister, Hannah Bondioli, tells what happens when they were called to their father's deathbed: "To me, he said simply, 'I love you.' To Emmie, he said, 'Promise me, you'll always take care of your sister.' I remember thinking, she already does."

Thus, much of the responsibility for running the household fell to her and, given the loss of the father's income, earning some of the family's income as well. Emmie played piano and organ at the community church beginning age 11, gave music lessons to other young people, started a church school and a music program at the elementary school and organized summer activities for the younger children in town. Resourceful? You bet.

It All Started with Lenny

By Ron Savage

President, Sarah Jane Brain Foundation; Chairman, International Pediatric Brain Injury Society; Board of Governors, International Brain Injury Association; Past Chairman, North American Brain Injury Society; Editor-in-Chief, Brain Injury Professional; President, The International Academy of Hope, New York City

For me, it all started with Lenny…

I was one of the many people in Rutland and around the state who watched Lenny's progress daily after his traumatic brain injury through newspaper articles and word-of-mouth accounts. Everyone who knew this remarkable young man realized early on that he was destined for great things. Lenny was smart, athletic, personable, mature, and caring. We knew all that about Lenny before his injury. What we didn't know was that Lenny, whose life would change so tragically in a brief moment of time, would also positively change the lives of many, many others.

While I had seen Lenny play basketball at Mount St Joseph Academy before his injury, I first met Lenny and his family after he returned from inpatient rehabilitation in California. Rutland had raised thousands of dollars to help support Lenny's rehabilitation. What none of us realized at the time was that brain injury rehabilitation facilities were very few and far between, and they cost an incredible amount of money. Even more important, we all thought after intensive rehabilitation that Lenny would return to Rutland "all better" and his life would go on as before. Yes, Lenny was out of coma, he was walking and talking, but he was not "all better." His life had permanently changed because of his traumatic brain injury.

I had been a special education teacher in the Rutland Public Schools when Lenny was injured. I had students with learning disabilities, attention deficits, and other problems, but I had never (or so I thought) worked with anyone who had a "traumatic brain injury." I now realize that many of my former students with learning problems had a history of brain injury, but at the time Lenny was an enigma to me. Shortly after I started a summer learning clinic at the College of St. Joseph, Emmie Burke contacted me to see if there were ways that I could help Lenny. I was both excited and intimidated by the request. What do I know about traumatic brain injury? What therapies will work for Lenny? What if I really mess up and make things worse?

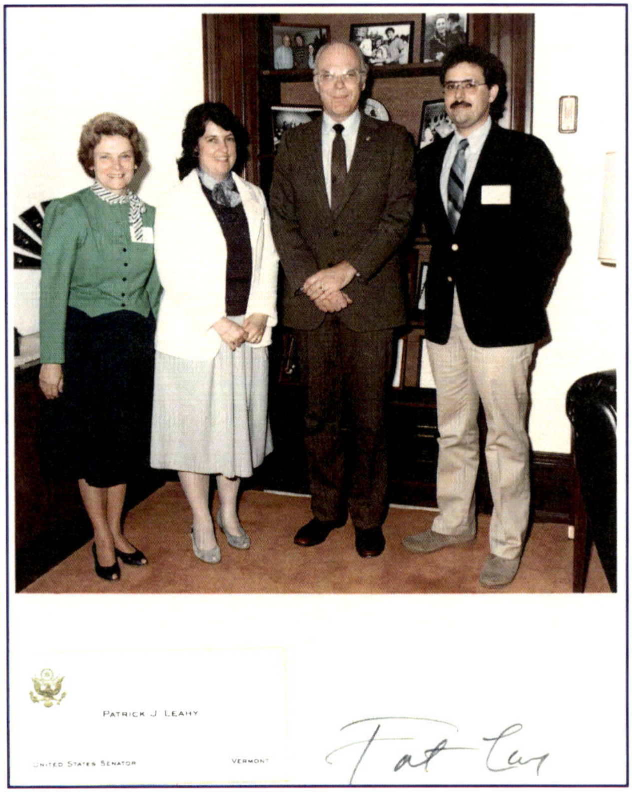

Marion Austin, Emmie Burke,
Sen. Patrick Leahy and Dr. Ron Savage.

Fortunately, Karlene Foy Marro was one of my graduate students in the Learning Clinic that summer and her insight into Lenny helped us to develop various therapies and learning strategies to help him with memory problems, attention and concentration problems, and problems self-monitoring his behaviors. Lenny and I continued to work together that following school year and developed more strategies he could use in his recovery. Lenny and I became good friends as well as "teacher-and-student." I remember bringing Lenny over to my house because my sons thought he was the "best basketball teacher in the world." My young sons did not care about Lenny's brain injury; for them it did not even exist. What existed was Lenny's joy in helping them make a jump shot or cross dribbling between their legs.

Rutlanders have hundreds of stories like this one.

Wonderful colleagues throughout Rutland helped Lenny and provided him opportunities to practice his "brain injury strategies" and to "get back into the game," not just basketball, but life itself. Slowly over the years, Lenny has improved his overall functioning which, in turn, has enhanced his quality of life. Frequently, when I was working with Lenny, people in Rutland would stop me and ask "How's Lenny doing?" and then they would always offer some other suggestions or opportunities for Lenny that were very helpful. Lenny had become a "team effort" in Rutland and people wrapped their arms around him in a hundred different ways.

Interestingly, what initially put me at ease when working with Lenny was certainly Lenny himself. Ever positive. Happy. Willing to try anything. Yet, there was also his mother, Emmie. To this day, Emmie Burke is one of the most remarkable, resourceful and intelligent people I have ever met. Her determination was unstoppable; her spirit was ever inspiring; and her courage was incredible. I knew that working with Lenny and his family would be an incredible experience and for me, ever the geeky guy, I knew I would learn so much.

Over the next several months working with Lenny, Emmie and I, along with others, wrote a grant to start what has now become the Vermont Brain Injury Association. Emmie used to say, "This is not just about Lenny. There are hundreds of other Vermonters in the same situation." Emmie always thought big. Nothing stopped her from dreaming, building, or creating. She was constantly asking questions to every professional she met. It did not matter who they were, physician, psychologist, speech therapist, Emmie would glean every bit of information she could and pull together the key elements. Emmie kept all of us searching and not becoming complacent with what we already knew (or thought we knew). It was Lenny who taught me about brain injury rehabilitation, but it was his mother who taught me to continually push forward to make the world a better place for people with brain injuries.

I have so many fond memories of working with Lenny and our friendship, memories that still endure today. I learned way more from him than he ever learned from me. For me, Lenny is and always will be my "Ground Zero." My career has been built around helping people with brain injuries and there isn't a thing I do and/or a new project I start that I don't have Lenny perched on my shoulder guiding me from afar. Lenny once said to me, "You know, Ron, a head injury is not a good thing to have, but it is not going to stop me. I have lots of things I'm going to do. You just watch." Prophetic? I think so. Lenny changed the world in so many little ways and made all of us better for it. I will forever be in his debt.

Later, when she was a mother herself, she continued some of these activities and also served as president of the local elementary school's parent-teacher organization. The community church where Emmie played piano and organ later became known as the Church of the Wildwood under the guidance of the Rev. Richard Marceau. Rev, as Marceau was known to his neighbors and parishioners, was like a second father to Lenny. That wasn't because Lenny was any more religious than any other young boy; to the contrary, although he was quiet and shy, Lenny loved a good practical joke and could be a bit impulsive. But he had a deep curiosity about human nature and from first meeting Rev would ask him questions that seemed beyond his years, questions about good and evil and heaven and hell.

While the church had long been known for its spirit of openness, under Rev's leadership it became even more ecumenical. Lenny came of age during the era of Civil Rights and the Vietnam War and like many in the congregation he wanted to discuss racism and the death of many young people, including residents of their own small town. Rev was the person to whom he brought these questions.

The church congregation grew during Rev's tenure, in part because he brought to these conversations his own experiences at war – he had served in the Korean War, a battle much like the Vietnam War for its lack of clear purpose other than to fight Communism abroad – as well as his deep commitment to ending persecution of people based on color, gender or creed. Beyond all that, Rev was an orator. He spoke like an average man, no fancy language, but his ability to use scripture as a way of opening up a dialogue about what was on people's minds in this time of change was quite effective. Rev had had his own struggles in life and understood the power of faith to change lives. He wasn't interested in blame. He believed in the intrinsic goodness of the human mind and spirit, volunteered at the local jail, and offered his services to those who were struggling with addiction. As a result, he and his wife Ellen were not seen as "religious figures," separate from the daily lives of people living in and around Chittenden and the other three churches where he served.

This may also have been because Rev had come to the ministry later in life, after serving in the military and working as a certified public accountant. Like Lenny and nearly everyone else, Rev had been particularly moved by Kennedy's assassination. In 1963, when Kennedy was killed, Rev had immediately gone in search of a church where he might pray; several were locked including the Catholic church he belonged to, but Rev found an open door at a Methodist church located near where he then lived and went in to sit quietly with his sorrow. That was the impetus for Rev deciding to become a minister himself and for him to be drawn to the Methodist church rather than the Catholic church in which he'd been raised. Besides, he was already a married man. No way was he giving up Ellen.

Even after the Burke family moved a little closer to Rutland, to the town of Mendon when Lenny was a sophomore in high school, Chittenden remained home. Emmie's mother, Dorothy Ormsbee, still lived in Chittenden in a house that Emmie returned to after her mother's death in 1993 and the kids spent as much time in the town as they did at home or at school, escaping to Chittenden Dam or one of their friend's homes as often as possible.

As the oldest child, Lenny set a high bar for his siblings. His grades were routinely among the top in his class, first at Barstow Memorial School in Chittenden and then at Mount St. Joseph Academy, and he excelled in nearly every sport. He was the quarterback on his high school football team and an above-average golf player. Basketball, however, was his obsession. He practiced by the hour, his progress followed closely by his parents and siblings, especially his father who shot hoops with him each evening after work. Emmie had already spent an hour or two shooting basketballs with him in the afternoon.

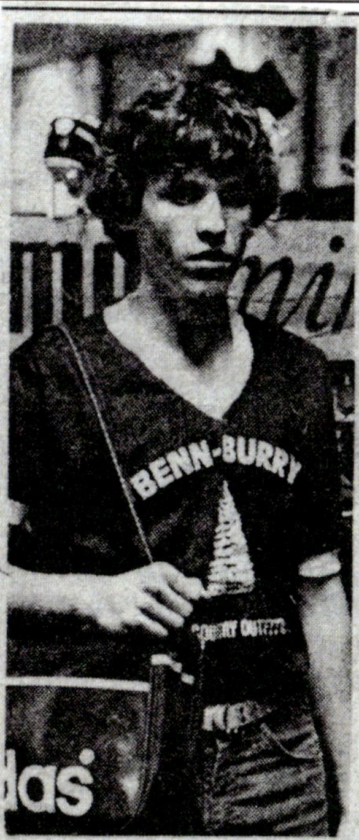

MSJ's Lenny Burke, the first winner in the Benn Burry 'Player of the Week' contest, poses on Thursday with a complimentary tee shirt and gym bag awarded him by the Rutland store. The Benn Burry shop will choose a local athlete weekly from MSJ, Rutland, Otter Valley, Mill River, Proctor or West Rutland high school to receive the award. Burke, a sharp-shooting guard, is averaging over 20 points a game for the Mountie varsity squad. (Photo by Drzewiczewski).

By junior year of high school, it was clear that Lenny was destined for college, perhaps with an Ivy League school and certainly with a sports scholarship. He was on the varsity basketball team at MSJ all through high school while keeping a straight-A average in his course work. He had a dream of playing college ball, then playing with his beloved Boston Celtics, and then a career as a medical doctor. It was a rather ambitious goal but Lenny had the goods, if not the imagination to envision such successes. After all, he'd accomplished much of what he'd set his mind to so far. He'd already received early acceptance to the University of Vermont and Middlebury College in their pre-med program.

During the winter season of his senior year, Lenny was the leading scorer in the Southern Vermont League and star forward on MSJ's varsity basketball team, well on his way to a high school total of 1,000 points. His stats were formidable: a 19-point average per game with 20 or more points in the three games leading up to a game held on January 23, 1979 when the MSJ Mounties faced rival Mount Anthony Union High School from Bennington in southern Vermont. The game was held at the Mounties' gymnasium on Convent Avenue in Rutland with what seemed like half the wider community in attendance. High school and college sports are still major sources of entertainment here in rural Vermont but this was true to an even greater degree in the late-1970s when Lenny was playing. Not only did many people in the community know the family but Lenny's aptitude on the court had received widespread attention in the local newspaper, the *Rutland Herald*, and rumors were that college scouts were attending the games.

On that fateful night, with only 5:15 minutes to play in the second period and a 20-15 lead, another MSJ player, Joe Kelly, stole the ball from an MAU player and threw it to the six-foot, one and a half-inch-tall Lenny. Lenny was having a great night with 13 points already. Fueled by the usual focus and determination he brought to his studies and athletics, Lenny went "coast to coast," as his guidance counselor David Wolk describes it, driving the ball down the court then rising into the air toward the basket for his signature layup. Lenny could jump high enough to get the ball over the rim. He was

Perseverance Furthers: Dick Bashaw

There's a trophy for fastest bicyclist that's been awarded for 33 years in Dick Bashaw's name at the annual Great Race Triathlon held in St. Albans. It's a bittersweet honor for Bashaw, once the second fastest bicyclist in Vermont. He sustained his head injury in 1984 at age 33 while bicycling home from a race he had just won. It was just the year before that he set the course record for fastest bicyclist, a record still not broken.

A passing motorist, perhaps misjudging how fast Bashaw was peddling, estimated at 35 mph, collided with him as the two turned onto the road to Bashaw's home. Bashaw was thrown 15 or 20 feet and landed on his head. His helmet smashed to smithereens.

Bashaw's injuries were substantial, both to his brain and to his body: his skull was crushed and he sustained broken bones and severe trauma to his brain, which caused some memory loss. But – and that is a giant but – he was determined to walk again and to compete again. And to return home to be near his family and friends. And to work again.

And it all happened, after he became the second client at Lenny Burke's Farm.

"Remember, Emmie," Bashaw said at a recent monthly social at the farm, "I'd have Wheatena for breakfast and Rev would say, 'What's that you're eating? Cement?' I always was into healthy living."

"My mother and I were praying we would meet one another, that there would be a place in Vermont for me to rehabilitate," he says, recalling how he came to the farm. At the time, Bashaw was receiving therapy at the Head Injury Center at Lewis Bay in Hyannis, Mass., a long drive from his parents' home in northwestern Vermont. They heard about Lenny Burke's Farm through the national brain-injury foundation.

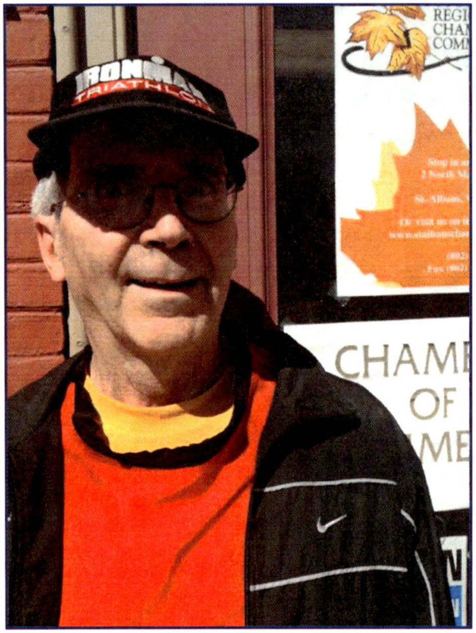

Dick Bashaw at this year's Great Race.

Bashaw's mother and brother fell in love with Lenny Burke's Farm their first visit, and when Bashaw came to try the place out, he told Emmie, "You feed me like this every day and I'll be one happy man."

Bashaw worked hard at the farm, fed the horses, helped with chores, and benefitted from therapy and treatment to repair painful hammertoes and other leg injuries that had kept him from being able to walk. He and Rev shared a love of the Bible and history, along with an equal devotion to good humor. They developed so many jokes about feet that Bashaw's podiatrist asked if he could use them in his public presentations, silly jokes that the two made up like: Why isn't your nose 12 inches long? Because then it would be a foot. Or, Why couldn't the two feet get along? Because they both thought they were right.

After several years of rehabilitation at the farm and later in a supervised apartment, Bashaw returned to St. Albans, where his brother Jim Bashaw had renovated a house he owned for him. He could no longer ride a bike, but he ran in road races for several years, competing in 25 five-kilometer races in Vermont and one in New York state one summer. He no longer can run but he participates each year in the St. Albans triathlon with a friend pushing his wheelchair.

Now 63, he will retire this June after working for 23 years as a janitor at the Bellows Free Academy.

Which is not to say that there haven't been disappointments. When Bashaw awoke from his coma, his younger brother Jim was by his side. That brother and his wife provided a stable environment living close by. But in 2000, Jim Bashaw got sick and died of brain cancer; both parents had also died. Asked how he was managing, he said, "I feel I have a hole that can never be filled up. The longer Jim's gone, the more I miss him."

But perseverance furthers and Bashaw has a strong support network in his community. These days, he works out on a Stairmaster every day. He still lives independently, and with the help of a life-skills aide his brother hired more than 20 years ago, Martha Dalton, travels monthly to Wallingford to attend the farm's social gatherings.

Says Emmie of him: "Without his parents trusting us with his care, we might not be here today. Dick came to us at a crucial time when we really needed another client. And, as with all our clients, he taught us so much.

"I was learning from him just as I learned from Lenny that by having a normal day, giving someone the opportunity to make their own breakfast, help them do their laundry, sit at a table with other people and have a normal conversation over a home-cooked meal, attending to their physical needs and creating a schedule for exercise and rehabilitation – all the things that we do every day in life – these were the keys to independence. Not everyone can get as far as Dick after a TBI, but everyone can have a good life."

"I know it's true," Bashaw says. "I'm living proof."

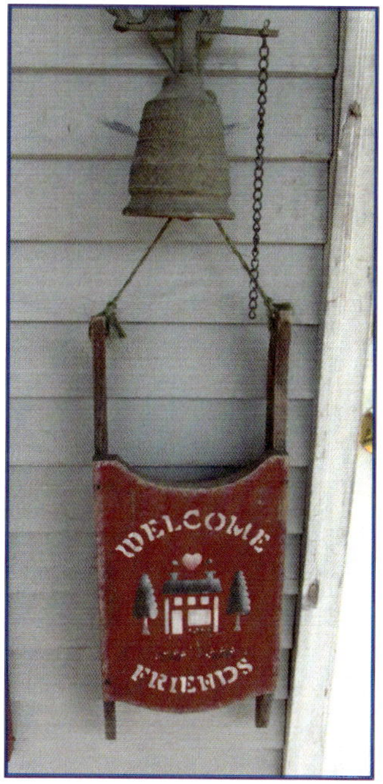

"Men ought to know that from nothing else but the brain come joys, delights, laughter and sports, and sorrows, griefs, despondency, and lamentations."

–Hippocrates

midair when MAU player Jim Cone undercut him, ramming into Lenny's legs and catapulting him against the backboard and then out of bounds with such force that Lenny bounced headfirst on the floor and then slammed against the wall located some three or four feet outside the out-of-bounds line. Like everyone else in the stands, his parents heard the sound of their son's head bouncing on the floorboards, not once but twice. Remarkably, Lenny was conscious for a few seconds. He even tried to stand up and continue the game before passing out.

That moment is as visceral to Lenny's siblings today as it was then. Kevin recalls the enormous collective moan of concern that swept over the gym. For Kathy, it's the sound of squeaking sneakers that haunts her to this day, that and the memory of the groan of apprehension and then the stone silence that filled the gymnasium as she and everyone else watched her big brother crumpled on the court.

"I ran down to the floor and the rest is a blur. I really thought that was it," Wolk recalls. In the stands, friends held Emmie back as Len raced to his son, helpless as the team physician Dr. William O'Rourke and Dr. Donald Wollins treated him on the floor. There was a cut under one eye and Lenny's neck was at a disturbing angle. Within minutes, Emmie convinced some strong men in the crowd to carry her son from the gym; she was afraid he had a broken neck. O'Rourke took over and Lenny was quickly transported to the hospital with his mom alone accompanying him in the ambulance. The game resumed but no one at least from the MSJ side was really paying attention.

That evening, former *Rutland Herald* sportswriter Carleton Laird wrote, "The MSJ players were overanxious to win the contest for their stricken teammate but a poor shot selection and several hurried shots did them in, despite a noble comeback effort." MAU won by one point, 50 – 49.

As Lenny's parents made their way to the hospital, Kevin went to the principal's office to call Michael, who wasn't at the game, and other relatives and close family friends. Gail Austin, the daughter of close family friends, Marion and John Austin, whom the Burkes had met at the Church of the Wildwood, quickly stepped in to care for Kathy, understanding the gravity of the situation and the fear that Kathy must have been feeling. This response was a precursor to the many ways in the days following the incident and the years from then to now that the Austins and countless other people would respond to Lenny's injuries. It was as if they all recognized this moment in time as pivotal not just in Lenny's life and that of his family but in theirs also.

The ride to the Rutland Hospital was grim, of course, with Lenny unconscious. But comfort awaited as the arriving ambulance was greeted by David Wolk. He had already called his father, Doctor Arthur Wolk, Rutland's favorite pediatrician who had treated Lenny since birth, and within minutes Doctor Wolk arrived at the hospital. O'Rourke had also contacted Dr. Peter Upton, Rutland's sole neurological specialist, and he too greeted Emmie and Lenny.

In small, tight-knit communities such as Chittenden and Rutland and long before Twitter and Instagram, news of the star player's injury spread quickly. Cone was charged with a flagrant foul and left the game but reports of the unsportsmanlike conduct of one MAU player and the resulting injury suffered by one of their own, the son of local residents, a kid with all the promise of a community focused upon him, soon garnered the sympathies of the entire community. Jim Kelley, the MSJ coach, ever the gentleman, came over after the game to talk to Cone. While he knew that the foul was the result of what MAU's coach described as Cone's "all-out all the time" competitiveness, Kelley knew Cone had not meant to hurt Lenny, just stop him.

Meanwhile, a drama to save Lenny's life was unfolding in the emergency room of the Rutland Hospital where Doctor Upton, himself a local hero for his dedication to his patients during the more than forty years that he practiced in Rutland, awaited the injured player. A standout athlete in high school who had been sidelined by his own sports injury, Doctor Upton had specialized in the fairly new area of medicine called neuroanatomy, the study of the brain and the nervous system, as a medical student at the University of Vermont.

While he could hold out little hope for the Burke family, recognizing the severity of their son's injury, Upton pledged to do all he could. Doctor Wolk proved to be invaluable as well. It happened that, because of the late hour, he was the only other physician in the small hospital at the time. Even though he had long practiced as a pediatrician and served as a medical doctor in World War II, Doctor Wolk had never assisted at a surgery. Yet, there was no time to wait for another doctor to arrive. Within minutes, he put on scrubs and was assisting Upton as Upton performed a more than two-hour operation to relieve the pressure of a huge subdural hematoma inside Lenny's head. Lenny was also started on a regimen of Manitol, a drug used to reduce intracranial pressure.

It was a long night for the Burke family who gathered together at the hospital and the team of players and coaches who joined them, a precursor to the longer weeks ahead. Upton had kept up with current events and discoveries on the treatment of traumatic brain injuries but the science was new and evolving. From the vantage point of what is known today about concussions, not to mention traumatic brain injuries, the understanding and treatment of serious injuries to the brain as recently as the late 1970s was quite rudimentary. The surgery to address the hematoma was a success in that it saved Lenny's life but Upton sensed that the damage to the young athlete's brain was severe. And there were other problematic injuries as well, especially the damage to Lenny's eye.

Upton and Wolk were the kind of doctors you read about – or ones you once read about before insurance companies mandated 20-minute treatment sessions. While both supported the family without giving false hope, independently they didn't even know if Lenny would survive and, if he did, what prospects for a normal life remained. Yet, they were both there at the hospital, day after day, hour after hour, as Lenny lay in a coma. Emmie Burke recalls Upton telling her, "I will treat Lenny as if he were my own son." Indeed, in the days and weeks ahead, Upton was known to tiptoe from his home late at night to check on Lenny through the hospital's back door so neither his wife nor his nursing staff could reprimand him for not getting enough sleep.

Beginning that first night, Emmie essentially moved into the hospital, setting up camp in the intensive care unit or in the nearby waiting room. After a few nights, she asked the other children if they felt neglected or found her absence too unsettling but to a one, Kevin, Michael and Kathy told her they wanted her to stay with Lenny. As Kathy put it, "If we were sick and in a strange bed in the hospital, we'd want you to be stay with us. We're okay." Len returned to work but spent his evenings at the hospital as well. He found, however, the prospects and worry about Lenny overwhelming and, unlike Emmie, felt useless and frustrated.

Fortunately, Emmie had lots of support, especially longtime friends such as Rev and Ellen Marceau, Dan and Claire Lawler, Marion and John Austin and Patty and Stuart St. Peter. Often, John Austin would sit with Lenny into the wee hours of the morning so Emmie could get a few hours' sleep.

Back at the Burke home, it seemed that Lenny's classmates needed one another. When they weren't outside the intensive care unit, the young people often gathered at the Burke home. There, David Wolk, the MSJ guidance counselor (who is now president of Vermont's Castleton State College), and his former wife Martha filled in as surrogate parents when Len and Emmie were away. This was a difficult time, of course, but David and Martha made the best of it, feeding and entertaining the children at home, playing endless board games and conundrums – logic and lateral thinking puzzles – driving the Burke children and whoever happened to be there to the hospital and to their own games and activities, trying to make life as normal as possible. Michael remembers that David Wolk even short-sheeted his bed one night.

Randy Tabor, Lenny's childhood friend, hunting and fishing buddy, was among the most faithful. Lenny had been the first friend Tabor made when he moved from Royalton to Chittenden and he took Lenny's injuries particularly hard.

Jim Kelley, Lenny's basketball coach, was at the hospital every day, too. He'd stand by Lenny's bed in the intensive care unit and review game strategy with the unconscious Lenny, asking for advice and discussing moves, just as he had before Lenny's injuries, treating him as if he were still the captain of the team. Indeed, as far as Jim Kelley was concerned, Lenny was the team captain more then than ever. And Lenny's teammates responded likewise with every game played for Lenny.

Emmie's mother Dorothy helped David and Martha Wolk and Len with the children. On the night of the accident, Emmie had asked Rev and Ellen to bring her mother to the hospital; she didn't want her mother to hear of the incident any other way. It wasn't until Emmie saw her mother that she finally cried that first night, but that was not something she did often. There were other reasons why Emmie wanted her very loving but sometimes unpredictable mother to hear the news from a reliable source, someone who would also deliver her to the hospital. In the following weeks, her mother could unintentionally add to Emmie's concerns as she heard stories about her mother hitchhiking to the hospital. Or she'd hear how her mother had tried to separate the boys and girls – half the MSJ student body – who had innocently fallen asleep on the Burkes' living room rug or in Lenny's room. Big Len's sister, Aunt Irene Vignoe, was another huge help, also quite adept at making sure the young people played by the rules. Dorothy, Irene and another family friend, Sue Klein, would meet in Lenny's empty bedroom every night at 8 p.m. and pray together. One night, Dorothy told Emmie she'd "gotten the message that Lenny was going to be alright." And of course, the Sisters of Saint Joseph said the rosary together for Lenny every night, with the locally famous Sister Clementine leading the prayers. It didn't matter that the Burkes were not Catholic. Emmie took much delight along with reassurance that the Catholics, Protestants and Jews were all praying for her son.

One of Lenny's closest friends, Jimmy O'Rourke, was particularly shaken by Lenny's injury. He came to the hospital every day and fretted that Lenny, so smart and athletic, the friend he golfed and played ball with endlessly, would be a vegetable. One day Emmie told him, "I promise you that won't happen. I promise you he will have a good life." As she said

AILY HERALD, WEDNESDAY MORNING, JANUARY 24, 1979

Mt. Anthony Nips Acads, 50-49

By CARLETON LAIRD

Sparked by Rick Pembroke's rebounding strength and game-high 18 points, Mt. Anthony held on to edge Mount St. Joseph 50-49 Tuesday in a Southern Vermont League game marred by the serious injury of MSJ's Lenny Burke.

Burke was injured with over five minutes remaining in the second period. (See story, Page 1.) The SVL's scoring leader had added 13 points and his absence was greatly felt by the Acads.

The Mounties were holding 20-15 lead at the 5:14 mark f the second when Burke eceived a long downcourt ass and was fouled by Jim one while airborne at- mpting a layup. Cone was ected from the game.

After Burke was carried m the gym the contest tinued in an atmosphere nificantly changed. The J players were overanx- to win the contest for r stricken teammate a poor shot selection several hurried shots hem in, despite a noble back effort.

Anthony roared back e a 24-22 lead and the eams entered the in- ssion deadlocked at

Parochials not only Burke's scoring but is board work. Im- tely after Burke's ure, Pembroke ran nt and tossed in eight before the halftime. eff Cushman points, broke basket, two hrows by Gerry and Gary Russ Mt. Anthony to a 36- at 5:27 of the third battled back.

Gilligan dropped in and a charity toss n Whittemore hit a from the top of the ut the margin to 5, but six straight s (five by Feenan) 2-35 after three.

he teams traded ps twice, Jim hit a foul ne nd later fed r a pretty hoo AU's lead to 4 ore they tr ut a raft of ats to the foul in the final 1:

Mounties, Mt. Anthony (which has been averaging nearly 70 percent from the line) was having difficulties from the charity stripe and missed all four opportunites.

With eight seconds to go, the Pats were whistled down for a traveling violation and MSJ got another run trailing 50-47. Whittemore came down the floor and did the only thing he could — go to the hoop in hopes of getting a foul and a three-point play chance.

Whittemore made the shot and got the foul — only it was on him and Russ went to the line shooting one-and-one with three seconds showing.

Russ' shot was off but the Mounties could only mangae a three-quarter-court, last-ditch effort by Whittemore which drifted way wide and the game ended with a one-point difference.

"This was our first win of the season on the road," said MAU coach Dave Fredrickson. "I wasn't particulary pleased but I guess it's nicer to develop experience winning rather than losing."

The win moves the Pats 3-2 in the league, 6-5 overall to while MSJ now stands at 2-3 and 7-4.

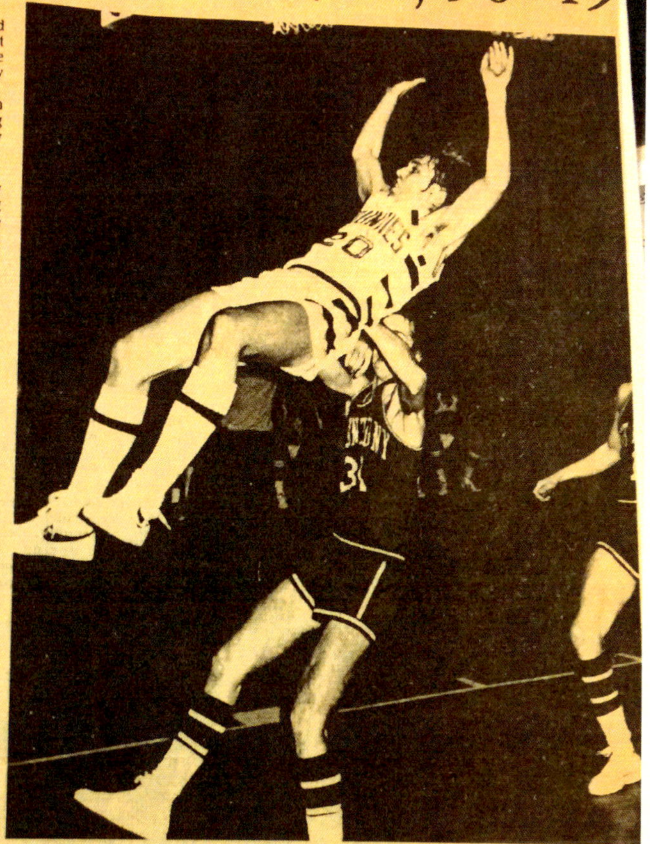

Len Burke of MSJ is fouled by Mt. Anthony's Jim Cone Tuesday night in a Southern Vermon League game. Burke was injured on the play and taken to the Rutland Hospital. (Photo by A. J Marro).

Injury

(Continued from Page One)

Burke, who had scored 13 points prior to the accident, still leads the SVL in scoring with a 19.0 average-per-game. The MSJ senior is a straight-A student at the Academy and has been playing varsity basketball for three years.

In league games this season Burke has contributed over 20 points on three occasions including 22 against Hartford and 26 versus Bellows Falls in winni causes and 24 points against Rutland i losing effort.

The Mounties' top scorer last seas Burke led the Acads to an 11-9 regul season mark and a class L playoff ber

Currently this season, MSJ stands at overall and 2-3 in the Southern Verm League.

The page one article following Lenny Burke's injury, *Rutland Herald*, Jan. 24, 1979.

those words, Emmie says, she knew they would come true.

Thus, in the weeks that followed, where there could have been chaos and disabling anxiety given the uncertainty of Lenny's recovery, a level of hope and solidarity developed among the young people, their parents, coaches, teachers and friends, and from this network grew other relationships that over time have led to a remarkable and sustaining future. Like Emmie and Lenny, none of these individuals knew then that together they were positioned at the bend in the road, one that would lead them not along the expected path, but to a future rife with uncertainties but new opportunities as well.

Because, such is life.

It's natural in a place like Rutland County that local folks would follow an injury like Lenny's and hang on to any development but it can't be stressed enough that Lenny was not just another kid in town. Only a few months previously, in his capacity as guidance director at MSJ, David Wolk had in a letter to admissions offices at a host of colleges in the Northeast described Lenny as "a rare breed." He praised Lenny's diligence and ambition, his success as the school's sole representative to Green Mountain Boys State, and his work as captain of the varsity basketball team where his teammates were inspired by "his quiet and determined leadership capabilities."

"Lenny has always looked for the best in others and given the best he has … Perhaps because of a strong and loving family background, Lenny has been resistant to negative peer pressures. Consequently, he has deservedly developed the deep respect of faculty and peers alike," Wolk wrote.

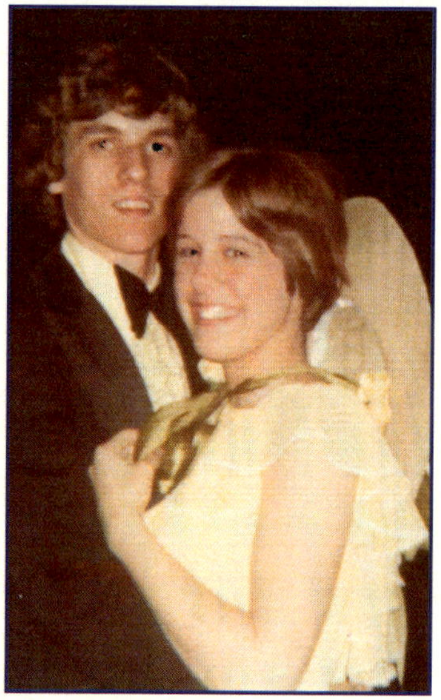

At the Cotillion Ball with a friend, Kathy Kantorski.

Perhaps more to the point, Pam Goddard, one of Lenny's female friends, noting also Lenny's looks, easy personality and the witty asides he was famous for – asides that kept him from being considered a goody-goody two shoes – recalls that at school, "Lenny was like a God." For Pam, like so many others, the reality that Lenny was near death seemed unthinkable. Yet, if the doctors were to be believed, it was a possibility.

In retrospect, Emmie's feelings were quite outside the norm. While she didn't want her son to die and wouldn't for an instant let herself believe he would, she wasn't afraid of that outcome. Indeed, she wasn't afraid of death itself. In explaining why not, she harkens back to an experience she herself had when she was a teenager just a few years younger than her son, a transformative experience she rarely speaks about but one that had left her with a lasting belief that death was not something to fear but rather a journey to a place of peace and reunion with those who, like her father, had "gone ahead."

This experience occurred when she just 16 and working for Sarah Baird, a Chittenden resident from a well-established local family who ran a guesthouse in the summer and fall. Emmie was in the kitchen when she suddenly fainted. Eventually, she was seen

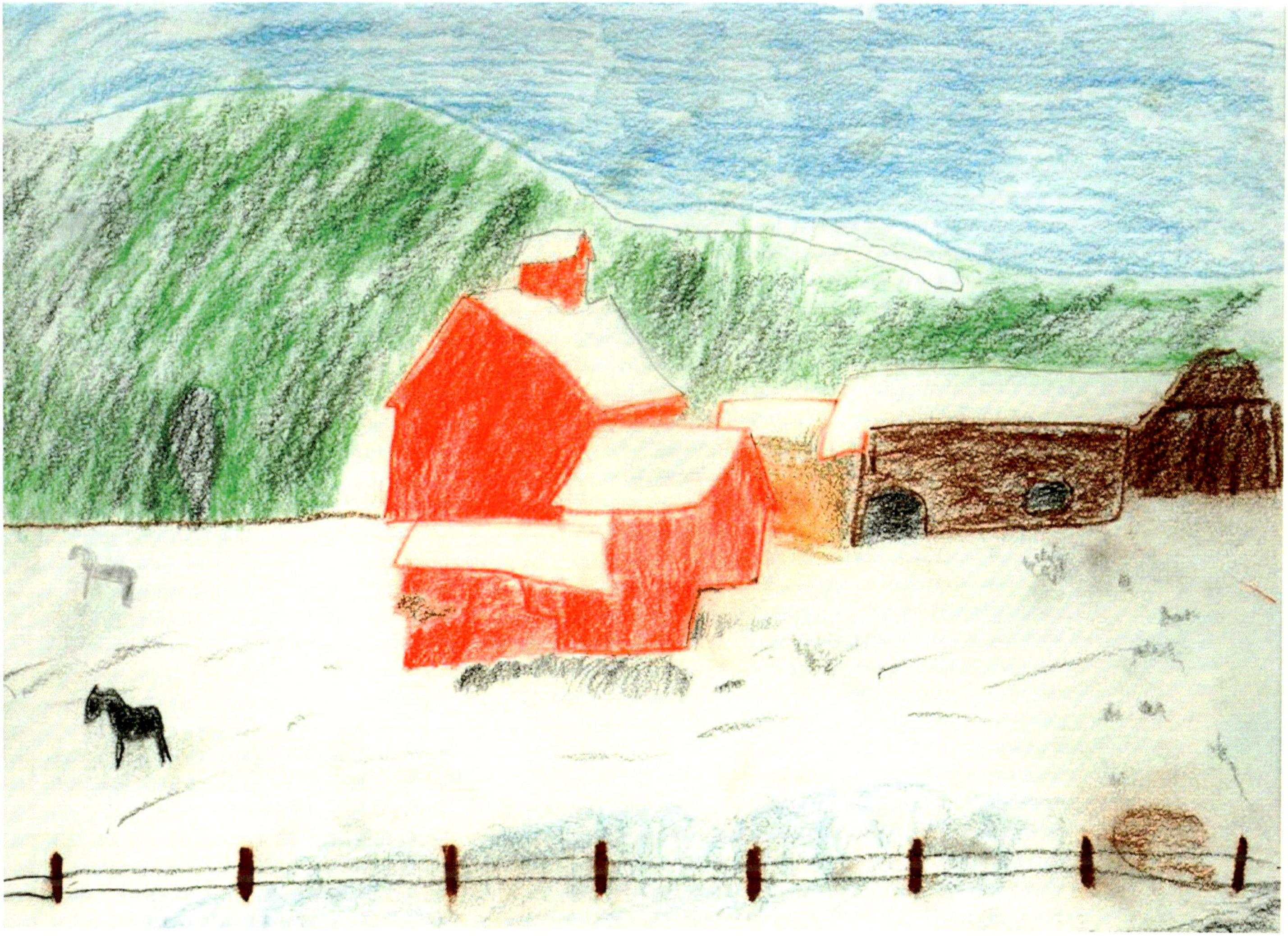

Both Emmie and Lenny imagined living on a farm where they could help people with head injuries. Lenny drew this picture of the farm he imagined about a year after his injury.

Meredith Coffey

Meredith Coffey was nine years old when a routine family trip for ice cream changed her life and that of her entire family. It was a Saturday, Sept. 11, 1993, and the America's Cup was in Newport, R.I., near where the family lived. They'd just eaten at a hamburger joint and were on their way for ice cream when a drunk driver slammed into her parents' car, injuring all six family members.

Coffey's parents and several siblings sustained injuries that required lengthy hospitalizations but hers were the most severe. An injury to her brain stem left her partially paralyzed and afflicted with a host of physical and mental disabilities. Her parents considered it a miracle when she came out of her 15-week coma on Christmas Day. But, says her mother, Diane Coffey, to a certain extent childhood ended for the Coffey children that day as the parents and children slowly recuperated from their own injuries while it became clear that Meredith's would be with her forever. She was in a rehabilitation hospital for thirteen months before returning home, where her mother became her primary caregiver.

In 1991 when Coffey was 17 years old, frustrated with the lack of appropriate rehabilitation programs in Rhode Island where the family lived and concerned that other services would disappear once Meredith turned 21, her parents brought her to live at Lenny Burke's Farm. She was Emmie Burke's youngest client, a girl with a most radiant smile, a smile that reflects her determination and resourcefulness. Emmie had to get a state waiver to take her because she was under 18 years old.

"When Meredith first came to the farm, no one thought she could do anything much for herself," says Kathy Chandler, who manages Emma's Place, one of the houses established for the cure of people with traumatic brain injuries. The girl had to be spoon-fed and needed help with daily care. Today, she lives in an adorable, flower-ringed cottage located on the grounds of Emma's Place, where she takes care of herself despite only partial use of one hand due to a serious tremor and weakness on her right side. She makes her own meals, keeps fit with a self-imposed exercise regiment, and follows advances in stem-cell research in the hope that her own injuries and that of others might some day be helped through science.

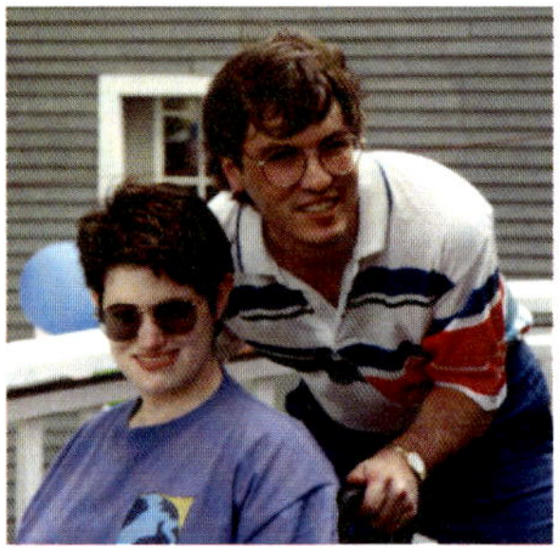

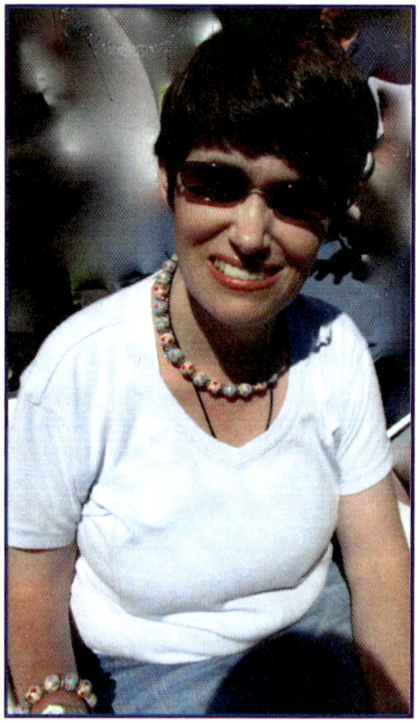

Lenny Burke and Meredith Coffey not long after she moved to Lenny Burke's Farm at 17 and Meredith today. "She does more with what she has than most people I've known in my life," Kathy Chandler, supervisor, Emma's Place.

"I get groceries for her but the rest she does on her own, just through sheer perseverance," says Chandler. "I find her amazing but Meredith doesn't think of it as amazing. That's true of a lot of these folks."

In an interview in 1991, three months after Meredith Coffey moved here, her mother said, "We knew almost immediately this was exactly what we were looking for. It's small, homey. The people are knowledgeable and very flexible, willing to try new things."

Before the accident, Coffey had been a typically energetic elementary school student, a tomboy whom

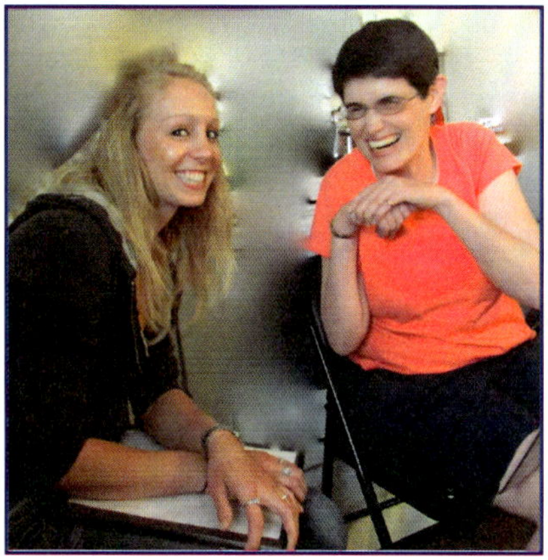

Life-skills aide Kayla Werner enjoys a joke with Meredith Coffey.

her father described as "fulla hell." Her mother had had a heck of a time persuading her to wait until the third day of second grade to wear her favorite camouflage outfit to class. Her daughter had joked that the teacher couldn't see her with it on.

The driver of the other car, Michael Faria, then 26, had spent the day drinking beer and champagne at the International Jumping Derby in Portsmouth, R.I., organized to raise money for the local chapter of the American Cancer Society. It was an unusually hot September day, over 100 degrees. Faria, driving a Chevelle SuperSport, crossed four lanes of highway before colliding with Neill Coffey's Rambler convertible. The vehicle's top was down.

Faria's blood alcohol count was .215. He served 18 months in jail but was allowed out of jail for daily work release. Two years ago, when he was charged with another DUI, the Coffey family's story again made the news. "All the anger my children had came back up," Diane Coffey says. "They lost their childhood back then."

Diane Coffey and her husband Neill formed the Newport (R.I.) Traumatic Brain Injury Association after their daughter's injury; Diane Coffey ran it for 10 years.

Today, Meredith can walk with the assistance of a specialized walking cane. She graduated from high school at 21, having received special services paid for by her home school district but supplied at the farm.

"She has made tremendous progress beyond what we were told to expect," her mother says. "She loves group and she loves Bingo because she wins. Still, she knows what she's missing. She wants to walk again, she wants a relationship, but given the degree of her injuries, she has had a wonderful life."

Her parents and siblings have remained involved in her life, talking on the phone every day as well as emailing regularly, and her parents drive to Vermont regularly to bring their daughter home for vacation. "I tell her she has the best of both worlds. When she's here, we have the ocean. In Vermont, she has the mountains. Yet, you still lie awake at night wondering what will happen when we're no longer there for her.

"What would we have done had we not found Lenny Burke's Farm?" Diane Coffey asks. "I don't know of any other program that's so caring and so good at meeting the needs of people in a positive way, of providing the feeling of warmth and home for people like my daughter."

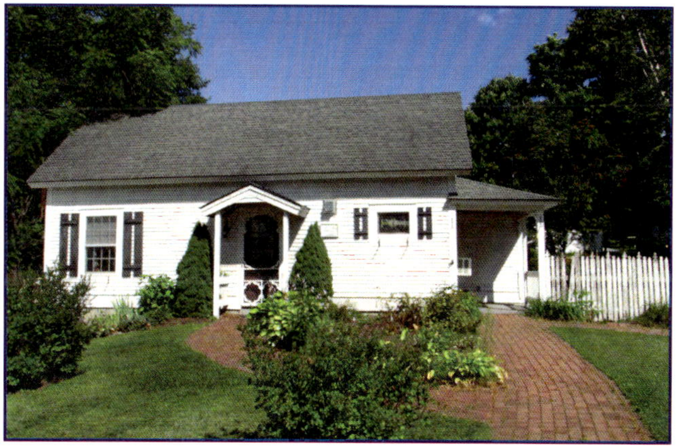

The sweet cottage that Meredith Coffey calls home. Living here, she is close to the other clients and staff at Lenny Burke's Farm but has the privacy and autonomy that she loves.

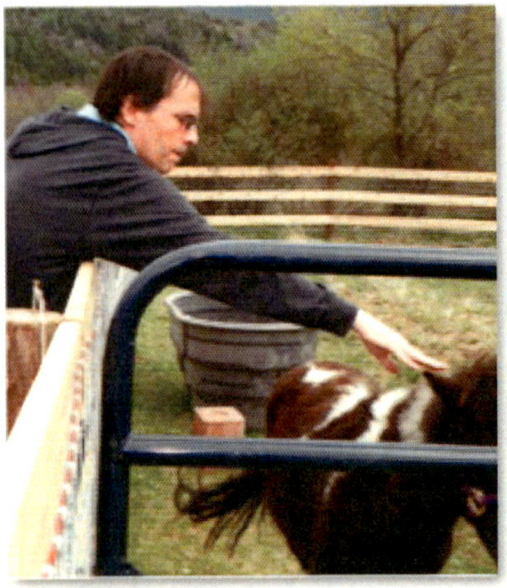

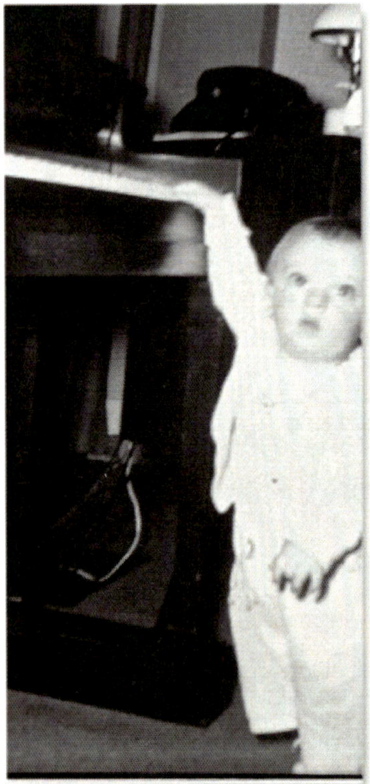

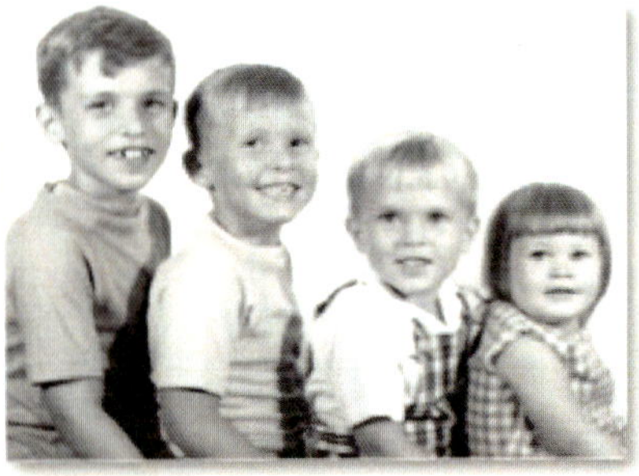

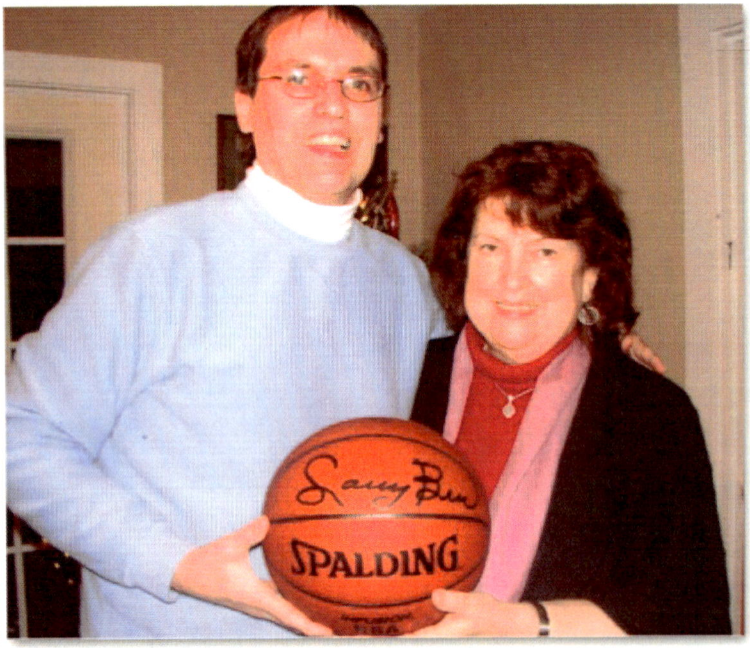

"I will never forget Lenny running up to us at Geno's wedding. He said, 'I just heard a great joke and have to tell it to you before I forget it,' which he did. Then with a sigh of relief, he said, 'Now in about 10 minutes, you can tell it to me, and it will be funny all over again. That's actually a fun part of this head trauma thing."

—Liz Pappas

"We are waiting for someone who will do it, but it's us."

—Ron Savage

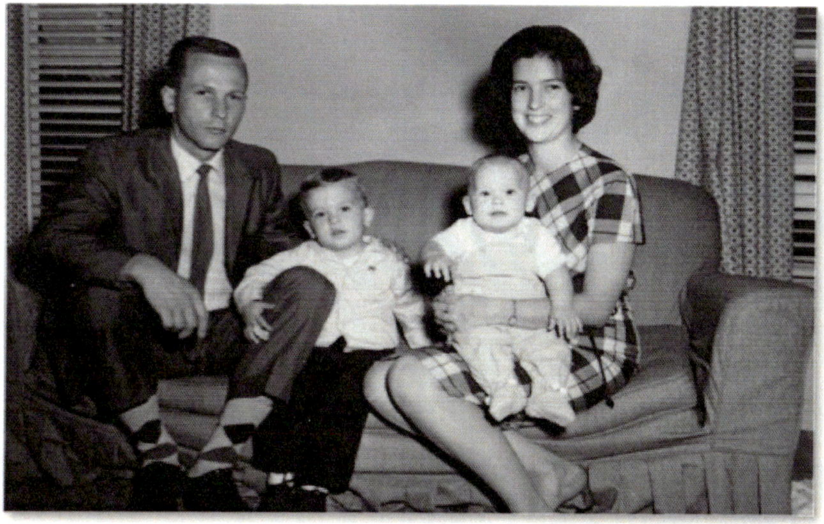

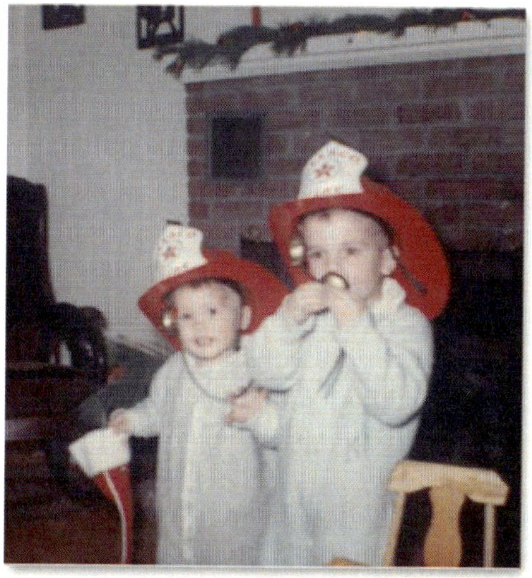

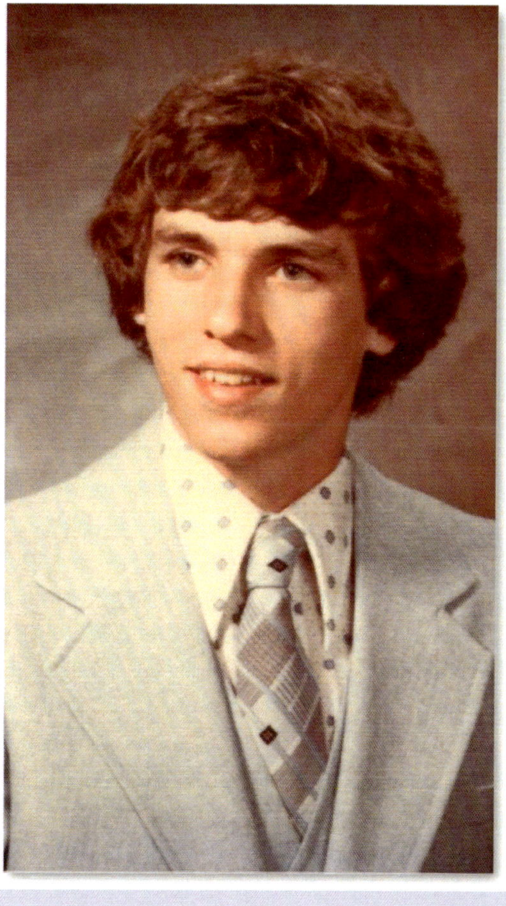

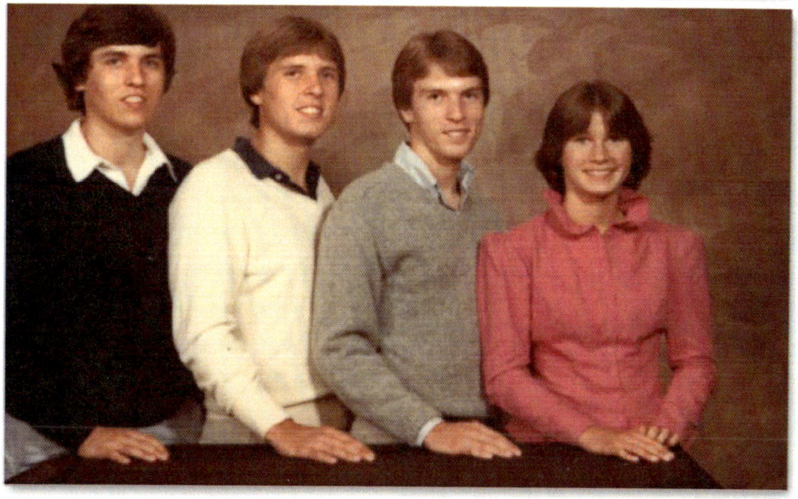

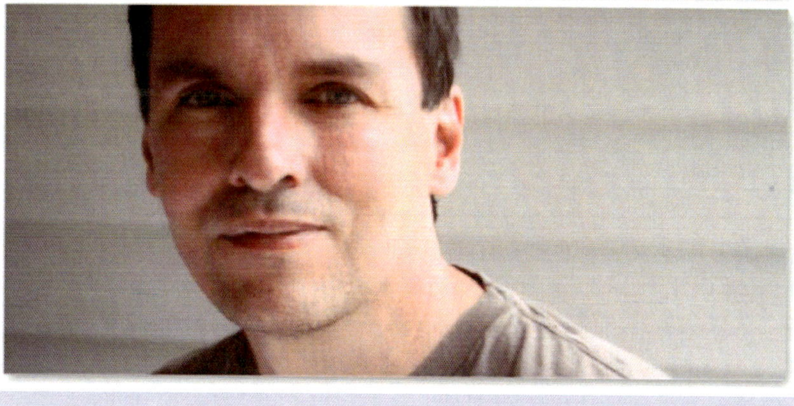

by the late Dr. Ernest Bove who discovered that she had a cyst on her ovary that needed to be removed.

The surgery was performed at the old Proctor Hospital, now a relic to changing times. It was a rather routine procedure that didn't cause much concern. Emmie was given sodium pentothal as a sedative but she had a rather dramatic reaction to the anesthesia, what she describes as being both alive and dying at the same time. To this day, she can recall the sense of separation she experienced, as if she were above herself, looking down at herself in the recovery room. She was quite aware that she was outside her body but she was not afraid. Unbeknownst to the doctor, she was allergic to the anesthesia. (Since then, she's discovered that her body over-reacts to some medicines, especially anesthesia.)

When she stopped breathing, she says she could hear and see Doctor Bove and his assistant in the recovery room reacting with fear and concern, trying to revive her with oxygen. "I was leaving – I could feel it – and enjoying the feeling. I was entering a beautiful light, suffused green color," Emmie recalls. Emmie's mother was brought in and the doctor told her that he could not revive her daughter. In response, Emmie's mom looked at her daughter and calmly said one word, an order, actually, in a firm but quiet voice.

"Breathe," she said.

Deep in her own state of unconsciousness, Emmie heard her mother's command … and breathed. But then she thought, maybe I don't want to breathe, this is awfully nice. Her mother said the word again, "Breathe," and Emmie obeyed.

"So when Lenny was in his coma, I told Dr. Wolk about my experience. I told him, 'I'm not worried about Lenny for himself. I'm worrying about losing him for me.' I told him I had faith and that I wasn't afraid of death, that I thought Lenny was in a safe place," she recalls.

Dr. Wolk had been a medic during World War II. He had seen some bad things. He was not a religious man. He told Emmie that day that he didn't believe in God. But while he didn't believe in God, he said his wife Florrie did, and he would ask her to pray for Lenny when he got home. He did and she did.

"I had faith in those prayers," Emmie recalls. "Dr. Upton couldn't understand it. 'Come back to reality,' he'd say. He didn't want me to get my hopes up."

Rather than pray, Emmie went into action, bringing her lifelong joy and passion for learning to the subject of brain injuries. She was appalled at how little there was to study. Before Lenny's injury, she had read an article in *Ladies Home Journal* about doctors experimenting with lowering the body's temperature and intentionally putting patients with severe brain trauma into even deeper comas so the brain could more easily heal. She kept asking Dr. Upton if he was doing these procedures. "Poor guy, he had to put up with me, right from day-one," she says. Meanwhile, Len was telling his wife to stay out of it, that the doctor knew what he was doing. Staying out of it was the last thing Emmie planned to do. A strength in her own convictions and power was growing and the last thing she was going to do was stay out of her son's treatment and, she was sure, recovery.

Dr. Upton had not heard about these new procedures and thought Emmie had read about them in a medical journal. When he learned the real source of the article, he and Emmie had a good laugh but the good doctor went home that night to discover the very same procedures outlined in the January issue of the *New England Journal of Medicine*. Because Emmie had understood the language (in the *Ladies Home Journal* story), Upton presumed she was a nurse or had some medical training. The next day he brought Emmie a copy of the *New England Journal of Medicine* article, which she could not begin to understand. More much needed laughter. Nonetheless, with little hope of it making a difference, Upton tried the procedures discussed in the article for the first time in his years of treating head injuries. Lenny had been injured on a Tuesday; Upton began the new procedures two days later, chemically inducing a deeper coma while keeping Lenny's body cool to allow his brain time to heal.

Meanwhile, another drama was unfolding, not just in the communities that claimed the Burkes as their own but in households throughout Vermont where the story garnered unusual attention. Along with the local news sources, the *Rutland Herald*, radio stations WSYB and WHWB, and television channel WCAX, the major wire services distributed updates on Lenny's condition. Inquiries about his condition poured in from around the nation. The switchboard at the Rutland Hospital was flooded with requests for information.

Rev was among those who spent hours at the hospital with the Burke family, talking to Lenny's teammates and teachers, and to his parents, offering whatever comfort he could. He also spent hours just talking to Lenny as he always had, usually beginning with his signature opening, "You know, I've been thinking …." At the hospital and at church, he cautioned those who cared about Lenny not to hate the other boy, the one who had caused such harm to Lenny, but to have faith that all things happened for a reason, even when we could not see what it was. He reminded them that that other boy was in pain too and that he had few people to support him in this difficult time, unlike Lenny. Even if the foul were intentional, surely Cone did not mean to hurt Lenny. He asked them to imagine how Cone was feeling as the story dominated the newspapers and the airwaves. He carried the message of the time: where there is love, there is hope. Blame does not help.

And love was abundant.

Another local man, Tied Levins, was in the hospital's intensive care unit in a bed beside Lenny. Even though the man was quite ill, he was alert. One afternoon into Lenny's second week of hospitalization, he told Emmie, "Lenny's coma's lightening up." He said Lenny had opened his eyes. He had heard the doctors talking about it and quite enthusiastically passed the information on to Emmie. Both Upton and an intensive care nurse, Kathleen Ledo, had seen Lenny open his eyes but neither took it as an overly positive sign nor were they anxious to share the information with Emmie. After all, Lenny had not spoken a word nor shown any other sign of recovery. Like Upton, Ledo told Emmie not to get too excited with the news. "Stay calm," she advised. They were well aware that people in vegetative states often have periods of eye opening and closing.

Calm? How could Emmie stay calm when her son had opened his eyes? Yes, he didn't seem to be tracking or making eye contact but open eyes had to be better than closed ones. "Everyone in the whole circle knew Lenny's eyes had opened up," Emmie recalls of the day that she heard the news; the circle was what they called the area outside the intensive care unit where the cadre of relatives and friends could be found at almost any hour of the day. "I'm in there by myself. I'm saying, 'Lenny I love you. Your eyes are opening up. You're getting better.' And all the while, Tied is yelling, 'I love you too, Lenny,' and everyone in the ward outside was shouting with joy.

"When Lenny opened his eyes in the intensive care unit, they were perfect. They were the eyes of a

"I have found home," Kathy Chandler

"I have found home. They'll never get rid of me," Kathy Chandler says of her job at Lenny Burke's Farm where she manages Emma's Place, works as a case manager for several clients living independently, and facilitates new clients' various medical, behavioral health and therapeutic services needs while also helping them adjust to the farm. And that's not mentioning paperwork.

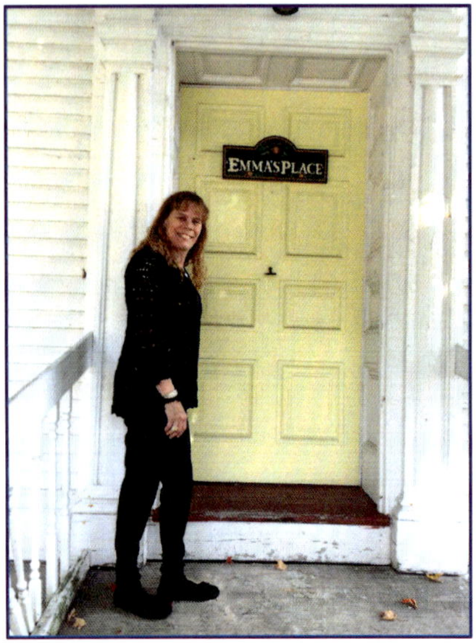

While that sounds like a formidable amount of work, Chandler says, "I'm used to a lot." Chandler sought out a job at the farm for a year before she was hired. She persisted because she understood that her philosophy about how to help people with disabilities was similar to that practiced at the farm.

It wasn't that Chandler's skills and work experience weren't ideal; just the timing wasn't. Chandler has worked with people with disabilities since she was 17, starting at the former Brandon Training School, then at Rutland Mental Health in outreach and crisis management from 1988 to 1994 when her daughter was born. In the mid- to late-1990s, she worked one on one in private therapeutic settings.

It was the arrival in May 2000 of Vanessa Doggett that created the need for someone like Chandler, who is trained in caring for a person with limited mobility who needs tube-feeding. It wasn't long before Chandler and Doggett were expanding Doggett's outlook on life with a new DynaVox communication system, an individualized exercise regime, and coordination of outside entertainment that included growing flowers and attending concerts by her favorite country western singer.

Kevin Burke notes that Chandler received the governor's outstanding employee award in 2007 in part because of her work in helping the facility grow in complexity in being able to care for and rehabilitate people with complex physical needs.

"This is the most real place I've ever worked. The quality of life for these clients is simply beyond anything they would have in any other setting," she says. "Everyone is moving ahead. It's a beautiful thing to be part of."

When Chandler talks about Doggett she realistically concedes that she still has "mountains to climb," but she says, "She's whole. She's loved. She's making a contribution. She's in a relationship. It makes me almost cry. Maybe in the end I see traumatic brain injury like dropping a mirror. At first you see all the broken pieces. Turn it a little to the light and you see all the colors. You look in one piece and you see the whole person, someone unique and special. That's what we're all about."

Chandler has also worked closely with another client, George "Geep" Parton III, a former food worker at Middlebury College who moved to Middlebury with his family in 1966 when his father became the college doctor. In 1998, he had a stroke. Parton lived alone and it was three days before co-workers worried when he didn't show up for work and checked on him. No one knows how long he'd been unconscious.

After hospitalization and rehabilitation, first at the Fletcher Allen Rehabilitation Center and later at Riverview, a rehabilitation center in Underhill, Vermont, Parton, now 63, moved to the farm. Following the farm's philosophy of building on a person's strengths rather than emphasizing limitations, it was apparent that Parton could eventually live on his own, with some oversight. He moved to a transition apartment about a few years after coming to the farm, and then about 10 years ago began living independently in an apartment house owned by Lenny Burke's Farm. Chandler assists him with shopping and communication, but he does his own cooking and travels by power scooter around Wallingford and to activities at Emma's Place.

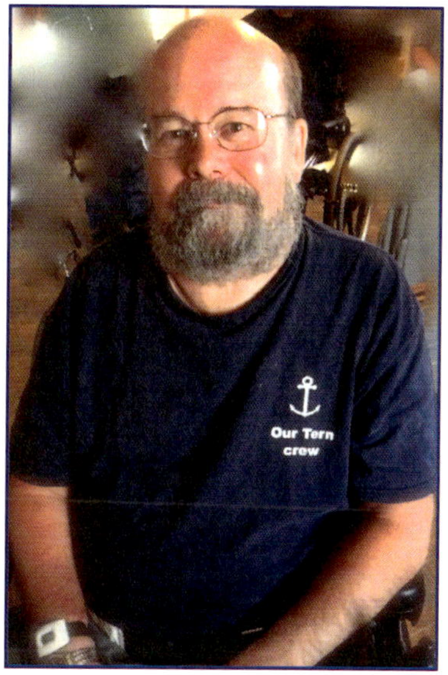

Because of the stroke, Parton suffers from what's called expressive aphasia, a condition wherein someone knows what he wants to say but can't get the words out. He has only a few words almost always said in doubles: yes, yes, good, good, yum yum, thank you, and ouy, ouy, which means something's making him unhappy.

To facilitate his desire for independence while acknowledging his limitations, Chandler developed memory tools for Parton that don't depend on speech. For example, he saves the labels from food he likes to help with his shopping list; he has photographs on his phone, which is programmed for both emergency and personal calls. He visits with his sister, Patty Paul, his two sons, Trevor and Evan, and Trevor's two children and Trevor's wife Becky regularly. And everyone involved in his care, along with family members, leaves messages and notes in a journal kept in his apartment.

Says Chandler of her life's work, "Each client is unique. I've discovered it's important to ask the right questions when you start rehab. We begin with where the client is strongest and build on that. Asking them to think of goals and building on them gives them a sense of ownership in their own recovery. Efficiency is doing things in the simplest way. Rehab is doing things right."

The last line is one you'll hear drop not just from Chandler's lips but also from others who have been working or living at the farm for years. It was a favorite quote of Rev's, the Reverend Richard Marceau, who co-directed the farm with Emmie in the early years.

Whether it's bringing in speech therapists to help with language development or physical therapists who specialize in some particular part of the body, such as the tongue, control of which is necessary so someone can speak and swallow, Chandler and the other staff members aim is to help each client live life as fully as possible.

As Parton's sister puts it, "Geep is living the way he wants to now, as much as possible, and he's content. Lenny Burke's Farm made that possible."

Brain injuries are most often caused by motor vehicle crashes, sports injuries, or simple falls on the playground, at work or in the home.

newborn," Emmie says. "It was as if he were seeing the world for the first time." Later, it became apparent that there was a serious injury to his left eye, which was quite deviated, as if the eye were off-center. And, even though his eyes were open, they weren't focusing on anyone or following movement, causing the ever-careful Dr. Upton to remind Emmie once again "not to get your hopes up."

When Rev came by just a little bit later and witnessed for himself that Lenny could open his eyes, he wanted to share what he had seen with everyone outside the intensive care unit. They already knew. That was how quickly and thoroughly news of Lenny Burke's health was followed and shared. No hashtags needed.

As the days unfolded, Upton became obsessed with measuring the cranial pressure in Lenny's brain, his only way of assessing if and when Lenny might die. Over the course of one day about two weeks after the injury, Upton measured the cranial pressure three times; it was high, high and even higher. He told Emmie and Len it was time to say goodbye. He didn't think the boy could survive much longer.

Each sibling recalls that day dramatically as they were pulled from school by their teachers and guidance counselors, and brought to the hospital to be with their parents. It was David Wolk who found Kevin between classes and drove him to the hospital, calmly inviting Kevin to play hooky with him. When they got to the hospital, though, Kevin saw his parents holding hands and walking the hallway in what he describes as "unimaginable grief." Seeing them, he thought the worst and was filled with gratitude that Wolk had brought him to be with Lenny and his family. To this day, Kevin recalls how helpless he felt, absolutely stunned with the thought that his big brother, the person he looked up to most in life, was about to die.

But then his mother took charge, as she had since the beginning.

Emmie remembered all the lessons she had taught her son and how he had passed them on to his siblings, how generous he'd been with his love for everyone, his remarkably positive nature, his athletic ability. She thought of her own out-of-body or near-death experience. She remembered the power of her mother's command: breathe. She thought about what the doctor had said about what would happen if the pressure in her son's brain didn't go down, not just brain damage and then death but gruesome realities as the brain's swelling pressed against the skull. She didn't want her son to suffer. If he were to die, she wanted him to know what a gift he had been to her and to so many others.

And so, she stood at his bedside. There were tubes coming out of her son and by now she could see that his eye was quite deviated. Martha Wolk had urged her to kiss Lenny's eye and she did. She kissed it to make it better, wishing that were possible. She believed he could hear her and so she held his hand and "told him all the things he had done in his life that I appreciated as he was growing up. How grateful I was for being his mother and sharing in all of his joy for each new season and what that would bring: winter ice hockey on Booth's Pond, skiing at High Pond; spring was always exciting as there was warmer weather; and basketball and then soccer was starting, but most of all school vacation for summer baseball, fishing in our back yard (and catching 56 trout in one summer), talking to our milkman and getting advice on trapping, swimming at the Chittenden Dam and Lake Dunmore, preparation for school and the excitement that he had for being with friends and learning more each year. I had so much to thank him for, the joy that he had brought into our lives and how proud I was for the man that he was becoming and the positive choices that he had made during his lifetime. It was the most difficult time of my life, but I told him I was going to 'fill him with love' and I was going to ask everyone to also do that. I told him if he lived, he might not be the same but I would promise him a good life."

"That night Kevin was waiting up for me when I got home – he was always quite protective of me – and I told him my plan to ask Dr. Upton to take Lenny off all of the medications and just let his strong vitals take over. I told him we would just fill Lenny with love and see what would happen. Kevin said simply, 'Mom, I'm glad *you* have a plan.'

"In the morning, I bumped into (Upton) in the hallway and he said, 'I am taking Lenny off all the medications and am just letting him fight this out on his own.' I will always remain grateful for the understanding that we shared for Lenny's care," Emmie says. She doesn't question the fact that they both arrived at the same conclusion at the same time. All these years later, she knows that something larger than her and Upton was going on.

Emmie instructed everyone waiting outside in the intensive care, the children, the little girlfriends and parents, Lenny's teachers and the nuns at MSJ to just "fill Lenny with love."

That day, Upton removed the gauge that measured cranial pressure from Lenny's brain. He took him off the medicines that he'd been pumping into his body and began to ready Lenny for a move out of the intensive care unit and into his own room where the family could be more comfortable in what he thought might be Lenny's last days.

Frank Bizarro, one of Lenny's other coaches, was among those who came to say goodbye to Lenny. An hour after leaving the hospital, he came back. He told Emmie he couldn't drive, that "something just came over me. I realized Lenny was going to get better and I had to come back and tell you that."

And, as Bizarro had predicted, Lenny did not die. The nurses, behind Dr. Upton's back, told Emmie that day that Upton had never been a believer in the power of prayer but now, one of them said, "He's becoming a believer."

One of the reasons for Dr. Upton's pessimism was that he couldn't get a good picture of what was going on in Lenny's brain because there was no CT-Scan (computed tomography) machine at the Rutland hospital. In the initial weeks, Lenny often ran a dangerously high fever and had a urinary tract infection. Once the fever was under control, Upton tried twice during the month of February to bring Lenny to the Burlington Medical Center in Burlington, 67 miles away. The medical center (now Fletcher Allen) was then the only Vermont hospital with a CT-Scan, but bad weather – snow and ice – prevented the trips. On the third occasion, Upton said, "I don't care what the weather does, we're going."

Emmie traveled in the ambulance with Lenny for the two-hour ride to Burlington. This was against protocol but Lenny had become quite agitated during the move to the ambulance and Emmie was the only person who could calm him. Once in Burlington, the CT-Scan showed exactly what Upton had warned the family about, dangerous swelling in the ventricles of the brain. Emmie and Lenny returned to Rutland with the bad news.

If Emmie had been the tiger mom, protecting her son from further harm before the CT-Scan, now she went on offense. Those tests didn't offer much hope but her gut told her something different; she believed that she and Lenny, along with others close to him, were in communication on some very basic

Advances in Treating Traumatic Brain Injuries

By Dr. Ron Savage

After Lenny sustained his TBI, many of us in the growing field of traumatic brain injury rehabilitation recognized that individuals with TBI needed more than just traditional rehabilitation therapies such as occupational therapy, speech therapy and physical therapy. It was, after all, the brain that was injured. That "thinking machine" that helps us pay attention, remember things, process complex information, organize our lives, and carry out plans. The "cognitive" part of TBI was being recognized by clinicians as a significant component in the rehabilitation of individuals after traumatic brain injuries. Today approximately 90 percent of rehabilitation facilities serving the needs of persons with brain injuries provide some form of cognitive rehabilitation, including combinations of individual, group and community based therapies.

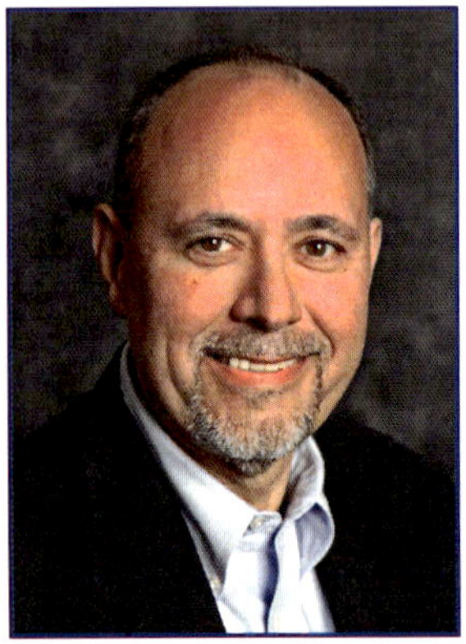

In the past decade, several groups have adopted cognitive rehabilitation treatment guidelines and position statements have been distributed by US and international organizations. In addition, the National Institutes of Health (NIH) "Report of the Consensus Development Conference on the Rehabilitation of Persons with Traumatic Brain Injury" (September 1999) concluded: "Evidence supports the use of certain cognitive and behavioral rehabilitation strategies for individuals with brain injury in particular circumstances. These interventions share certain characteristics in that they are structured, systematic, goal-directed, and individualized and they involve learning, practice, social contact, and a relevant context."

Unfortunately, in the United States, it is often difficult for clinicians to get paid for providing cognitive rehabilitation services to individuals with brain injuries. For example, Blue Cross and Blue Shield reported in 2004 that "The efficacy of cognitive rehabilitation has not been adequately demonstrated; therefore, cognitive rehabilitation does not meet the criteria for covered services." More recently, however, an independent external review organization overturned a BlueCross BlueShield of Montana denial for cognitive rehabilitation services, requiring the company to pay for treatment after a year of denials and appeals. Not long ago, Aetna also reversed its previously restrictive policy and now states "Aetna considers cognitive rehabilitation as adjunctive treatment of cognitive deficits (e.g., attention, language, memory, reasoning, executive functions, problem solving, and visual processing) medically necessary…" as long as the deficits were acquired from a neurological event, the individual has been properly evaluated (medical and neuropsychological), and the individual is expected to make significant cognitive improvement. Such recognition of the importance of cognitive rehabilitation did not come easily and much still remains to be accomplished.

Since I started working with Lenny, the practice of cognitive rehabilitation has changed substantially to the benefit of both practicing clinicians and individuals with brain injuries. There is still much work to do, but the foundation has certainly been established.

Jim Fleshman: Born to Ride

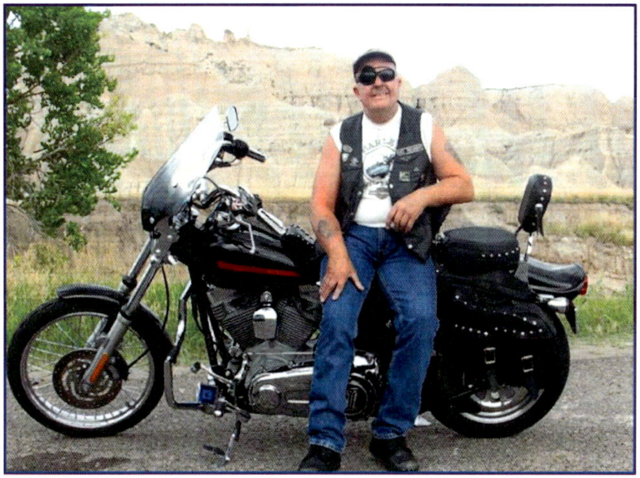

Jim Fleshman says Richard Keane, director of Serenity House, gave him back his life and the Lenny Burke's Farm helped him live it in a way he could not have imagined 20 years ago when he was struck by a hit-and-run driver. Here he is on his motorcycle in the Badlands on his cross-country motorcycle trip to Sturgis, South Dakota.

Jim Fleshman's story will resonate with those who have struggled with alcohol addiction and those whose loved ones have faced similar battles. Fleshman, originally from Albany, NY, was one of those kids who would try just about anything. He thinks his father's death when he was 16 may have set him on a reckless path. That's not unusual for young people who experience a close death; inexplicably, that kind of trauma sometimes makes young people try to defy death.

One day, he and four of his friends climbed an electric pole to the top, a typical teenage "look at me" daredevil act, only Fleshman slipped, touching the wire. About 225,00 volts of electricity went through his body, and he fell. His head was split open and his body was badly burned but, while two of his friends went to get help, he got up and ran away, afraid to get in trouble. He was hospitalized for more than a month.

The alcohol came later, the usual saga: drunk driving and the loss of his license, drugs, tickets, fights. He escaped to Bennington, where he had a girlfriend and got a new job. He worked as a mason, hard work that left a man thirsty. And so, the alcohol came too, and the girlfriend eventually kicked him out and took the car keys away. She went so far as to pull the wires from her car. He walked to where he could get a drink, and that's where the second head injury occurred, a hit and run in Shaftsbury on July 2, 1994.

The accident was all over the news and, as the driver cleaned up the car and removed the damaged windshield, someone who had read the story became suspicious and called the police. Fleshman's DNA was on the fender but, while the driver was prosecuted, he, too, had no license and no insurance. Fleshman was in a coma at the Albany Medical Center for three weeks and remained there for another two and a half months, whereupon no one seemed to know what to do with him. He had memory problems and a body that didn't work right anymore. He was just 28 years old.

Fortunately, his last address had been in Vermont and Vermont Medicaid picked him up. He was transferred to the Rutland Hospital where he was evaluated and given some therapy, but he was talking crazy stuff and really just wanted to go back to using again. There was talk of sending him to the state mental hospital. Enter Richard Keane, himself an alcoholic, long sober, who is now the director of Serenity House, a substance-abuse treatment and rehabilitation center, located in Wallingford not far from Lenny Burke's Farm.

Keane told the doctors Fleshman wasn't crazy; he was suffering from years of abuse and needed help of a different kind.

"I just didn't know stopping could be part of my recovery. My brother had told me, 'You're in Vermont; stay there,'" Fleshman recalls. But unlike the brother, Keane didn't give up on him; he simply moved him to Serenity House. Fleshman puts it simply, "Richard Keane saved my life."

Initially, Fleshman couldn't walk at all; his right leg "was a mess" and his right arm stuck out at an angle. But he was determined to get better. He worked out and did his exercises. He went to meetings. He got healthy and progressed from the wheelchair to a walker.

That's when he heard about Lenny Burke's Farm. Emmie agreed to take him as a client for a trial week after his sobriety was secure and, when a bed became available, Fleshman took it rather than move to the Bardwell House, where he also had been offered housing.

"Second best move I've ever made," he says.

Keane or someone else would come and pick him up at the farm and take him to meetings. He called the vehicle they used the druggie buggie. "I said, one day, I'm going to drive this thing."

He was like no other client. "Jim Fleshman wanted to do everything yesterday; he wanted to get better yesterday," Emmie says, recalling how hard he worked. Rev took an interest in him and with Len Burke, Sr., built wheels like training wheels taken from a baby carriage for his motorcycle so Fleshman could regain his balance. He practiced with them for hours at a time.

"I didn't like needing help," he says. "I had to get someone to help me go to the bathroom. I wanted to do it by myself. The same with making a bed or taking a shower. I just kept at it until I could do the thing for myself. But I owe it all to being clean and sober and the support everyone here gave me."

Eventually, Emmie came to Fleshman with a question: How would you like to get your own apartment? He was among the first clients to move into one of the farm's supervised apartments; it was across from Sal's restaurant in downtown Wallingford, and he lived there for a year and a half before he was able to get a place on his own.

Early on, Fleshman wanted a job at the farm. Rev gave him one cutting the grass. He needed a cane to get on the tractor but it gave him a sense of giving back.

One day, he got too close to the river bank and the tractor flipped.

"I ended up in the creek. I somehow got back up and to the office, half crawling and all muddy. Rev goes, 'Are you alright?' 'I am,' I say, 'but I don't know about the tractor.' 'Don't worry about the tractor. Tractor's can be replaced; you can't,' he told me. That's Rev, alright. You first. I miss him like there's no tomorrow."

Remember the druggie buggie? One of the obstacles Fleshman faced in getting his license back was his vision. His head had gone through that driver's windshield, smashing his right eye socket and leaving him with double vision. After 11 operations, doctors discovered that the other eye had perfect vision and that, with a patch on the bad eye, he could see fine. "The patch is better than another surgery," says Fleshman.

Meanwhile, Jim Kelley, Lenny's former basketball coach who was also a driving instructor, gave Fleshman lessons and he got his license back and he became one of the guys who picked people up for meetings in the druggie buggie. And, eventually, he was able to get back on his Harley and ride.

For years now, Fleshman, now 49, has given back to the Lenny Burke Farm, working as a life-skills aide and "doing whatever needs to be done." He loves to ride his Harley accompanied by his girlfriend Rachel whose Harley is "better than his," harvests food from his own garden at the home he owns in West Rutland.

As Rev had done with him, Fleshman took an interest in Jason O'Connor, a client who loves music, especially heavy-metal, and together they have been to a lot of concerts, all metal bands: Plant and Page, AC/DC, the Oz Fest, Iron Maiden, Judas Priest, Black Sabbath. "I love that kind of music, too," Fleshman says.

He volunteers with Vermont Adaptive Ski and Sports programs, where he helps brain-injured and autistic kids learn how to ski, and, also, at the Gymnasium, where he enjoys working with kids who have challenges that he can relate to.

"Life's good," Fleshman says. "Everybody tells me at the gym, write a book about your life. I tell them, I lived it. I survived. I'm just glad to be alive."

Traumatic Brain Injury (TBI) is the leading cause of death and disability in children and adults from ages 1 to 44.

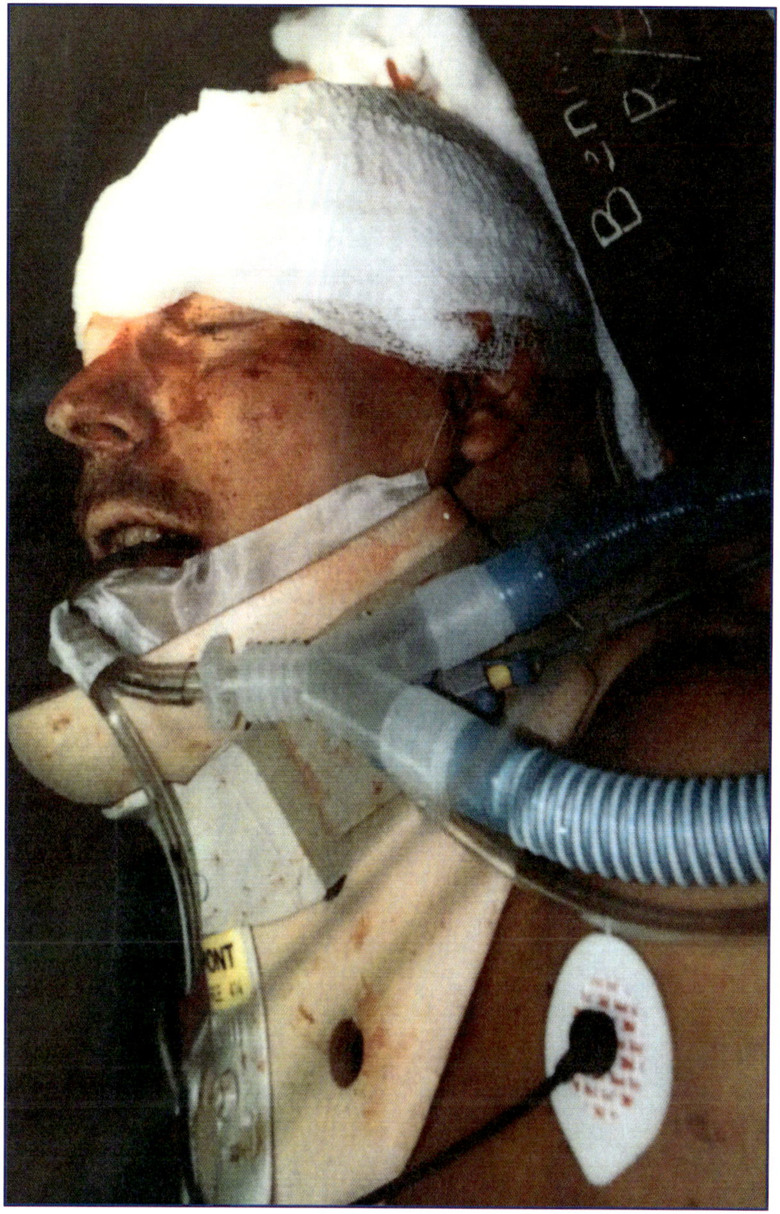

It's not a pretty picture: Jim Fleshman after his accident in 1994. Today, he gives back to the communities that helped him get sober and regain his independence after a traumatic brain injury. Fleshman uses this photo when he talks publicly about drunken driving and the dangers of traumatic brain injuries.

level. She was constantly frustrated that there wasn't more information available to parents and other individuals like her who wanted to understand the workings of the brain after a severe injury. Emmie's review of the literature at hand revealed that most people either lived or died with little medical intervention and of those who survived many remained in vegetative states. With little to go on, she went on instinct. She had heard or read somewhere – thank goodness she was an avid reader with a good memory, even if some of that reading was women's magazines – that the sense of smell was the oldest of the human's senses and the last to go, even in the case of severe trauma to the brain.

If this were so, why not try to reach her son through the sense of smell? It couldn't do any harm. With the freedom that came with a private room rather than the more restricted intensive care unit, she went home and dug out Lenny's smelly sneakers – the ones she'd threatened dozens of times to throw away – and hung them over his bed so they were near his nose in the hospital room. She doused him with her favorite perfume and his father's after-shave cologne. She waved his girlfriend's perfume under his nose.

She tried to reach him with the other senses, too. She ate pizza, Lenny's favorite food, sitting on the side of his bed, chewing loudly and describing in vivid detail how good it tasted. She kept the television or radio on for hours at a time, especially if Jack Healey was broadcasting an MSJ game. Was it her imagination or did Lenny seem to perspire when the score got close or MSJ was behind?

She knew her son, a typical teenager. What was one of the things he wanted most? The car keys, of course! She shook them in front of his face. She placed them in the right-hand pocket of his football jacket, which she held up over his bed. She told him where the keys were and asked him to find them. He did. One day a nurse placed a popsicle in Lenny's hand rather than holding it to his mouth as had been her routine, allowing the melting liquid to refresh his mouth and throat. Lenny held it on his own. Jokingly, the nurse said, "Okay, Lenny, now let's see *you* brush your teeth." Rather than brush his teeth for him as she had occasionally done, she placed a toothbrush in his hand. Remarkably, Lenny began brushing his teeth, adjusting the brush's angle as he moved it from one side of his mouth to the other.

Dr. Upton had developed a routine of stopping by each evening to ask Emmie in a half-teasing tone, "Well, what did Lenny do today?" That night, Emmie said, "Well, he brushed his teeth." Upton was skeptical but then he witnessed Lenny brushing his teeth the way the nurse and Emmie had described. Without offering a reaction as to what he thought about this, Upton just walked around the room, saying over and over as if thinking out loud, "So, Lenny brushed his teeth."

Says Emmie, "Maybe he *was* beginning to believe."

Soon after the accident a committee was formed with John Austin, attorney J. Fred Carbine, Jr., Rutland Mayor Gilbert Godnick and numerous others working together to raise funds to help the Burke family. If Rev, Doctors Wolk and Upton were institutions in Rutland County, so too were Carbine and Godnick, big men with big personalities who got things done whether it was in the courtroom or city hall. Their idea was to hold a two-day fund drive they would call "Lenny Burke Days" to be held on March 9 and 10, a month and a half after Lenny's injuries and, by chance, just one day after the trip to Burlington. Lenny had been in a coma for 45 days by then.

It was clear to these individuals that even if Lenny were to regain consciousness, his injuries would require expensive medical care. While no one knew what all this might entail, these local men knew that money would be needed, not just for Lenny's care but perhaps – hopefully – for rehabilitation.

On March 9 and 10, a Friday and Saturday, local radio stations WHWB and WSYB conducted radio-broadcasted fundraisers held at the Mount St. Joseph gym with Jack Healey, the voice of local sports, on the air broadcasting a play by play narrative as donations came in. Committee members hoped the drive would raise $20,000 to $30,000 but within a few hours after the campaign began, more than $10,000 had already been raised. By the weekend's end, more than $60,000 – equal today to about $180,000 – was donated.

For the fundraisers, it was another lesson in community. One man came in and asked if they could cash his welfare check of $84. He told Carbine, "Give me six bucks back. I'll eat peanut butter for two weeks." When all the donations were counted, including those sent in by mail, some from far-distant locations, or hand-delivered over the next few days, the total was $90,000, equivalent to roughly $270,000 today. It was the most successful fund-drive in Rutland history.

Dr. Upton may have been a realist but he wasn't giving up on Lenny either. And thus, on the first day of the fundraiser, he tried one more thing. Now that Lenny's infections had cleared up and he had a clear picture of what was going on in Lenny's head, he inserted a ventriculoperitoneal shunt into the young athlete's brain, hoping to drain excess fluid from the ventricles of his brain to reduce swelling. There were dangers with this procedure as well, not just the risk with any operation – the cerebral shunt went into a ventricle of the brain and connected to a tube that went behind Lenny's ear and drained into his abdominal cavity – but Upton knew the procedure could also cause a blood clot or exacerbate the bleeding in the brain. It could bring on seizures or cause an infection in the brain or throughout his body. The night before the surgery, Upton urged Emmie not to have false hope in the procedure. "I don't want you to be heartbroken," he said. Emmie took Lenny's right hand in hers and began to cry. But then, Lenny brought her hand to his lips and kissed it. She knew his vital signs had remained strong throughout the ordeal and that he had never stopped breathing. His brain had never been without oxygen. She took the kiss, like the kiss she'd given him on his eye a few weeks previously, as a sign.

"Lenny is in there," she thought.

On March 9, as the fund drive ensued, Upton was in the surgery room inserting the shunt into Lenny's brain. The radio had been on all day. Like everyone else, Upton talked to Lenny as if he could hear him. As the excited announcements came blasting out from the radio, Jack Healey's familiar voice keeping the tally much as he did night after night keeping the score of local sports games, Upton said quite casually, "You hear that, Lenny?"

And from Lenny's mouth came these words: "I hear that."

An astonished Dr. Upton didn't tell Emmie right away that Lenny had spoken. Again, caution prevented him from putting too much stock in three words. However, when Emmie stepped into Lenny's room later that day, her son quite matter-of-factly asked her for a glass of water. "I hugged him and screamed and hollered," she recalls. She called everyone then went home to tell the kids. By morning, Upton had been back to the hospital and realized that the sentence he'd heard was not a fluke; Lenny was actually talking quite a bit. And not just

Therapy Is Freedom

By Gary Miller-Wade
Life-skills aide and group meeting director, Lenny Burke's Farm

We have seen many examples of the power of music performance on rehabilitation therapy at Lenny Burke's Farm. A large audience is not necessary, a small circle of friends is all that is needed. It is the enthusiasm of the group that is important. And there is power and freedom in the group.

Once the song comes out of your mouth all other thoughts quickly vanish. The entire brain is working on the song: the lyrics, the melody, the rhythm and the cadence. The lungs are working to keep the breath that pushes out the words and notes. The annunciation of lyrics exercises the mouth and throat and sends this information back to the brain to be used again later. The feet are tapping or the hands are clapping, exercising and stimulating the brain-muscle connections. The brain's pleasure centers are reacting. There is so much going on, that there is little chance to think about anything else, including problems.

Music just makes you feel good when you're singing along with your friends. At our weekly Thursday afternoon gatherings at Emma's Place we have witnessed improvements in annunciation, articulation and projection of voice and speech. We have seen confidence built, which carries over outside of the group. We have seen people slowly come out of their depression and loneliness so often evident on the path to recovery. There is freedom in the music. Like a river flowing. It's a therapy. You don't need to do anything but enjoy it. Sing along!

The Power of Song

The song, "American Pie" has so many complicated stanzas that it takes up three pages in the songbook that clients and staff use during Thursday group meetings at Lenny Burke's Farm. A few groans rise up when one of the clients requests it, mostly from the staff. The clients are up for the challenge. Gary Miller-Wade, who leads the Thursday group sessions and sing-along and also works as a one-on-one aide to one of the clients, quickly quips, "We do all the requests here at WADE radio."

And before long, everyone is singing, "Do you believe in rock 'n' roll? Can music save your mortal soul?"

It's almost unbelievable to watch clients who can only say a few words – fellows like George Parton, aka "Geep," whose vocabulary usually includes only yes, good, thank you, and aiii, aiii, aiii, which means something is making him unhappy – singing stanza after stanza of this and some 20 other songs on a given afternoon.

Everyone has a favorite. "Cotton Fields" for Meredith Coffey; "Country Roads" for Jean McDuff; "You're Time is Gonna' Come" for Jason O'Connor. There's joy in the room as the words spill forth, old favorites like "King of the Road" for Daniel Patrick Fanning, for whom they also always sing, "Danny Boy," and "Will the Circle Be Unbroken" for the Rev. Richard Marceau, the man the clients who knew him never forget. In a beautiful way, Rev is there in each Thursday's sing-along.

Miller-Wade is on guitar, making the rounds, stopping in front of Erich "Buddy" McLellan to sing directly to him, leaning in close and pausing while McLellan, his voice barely audible, sings the next

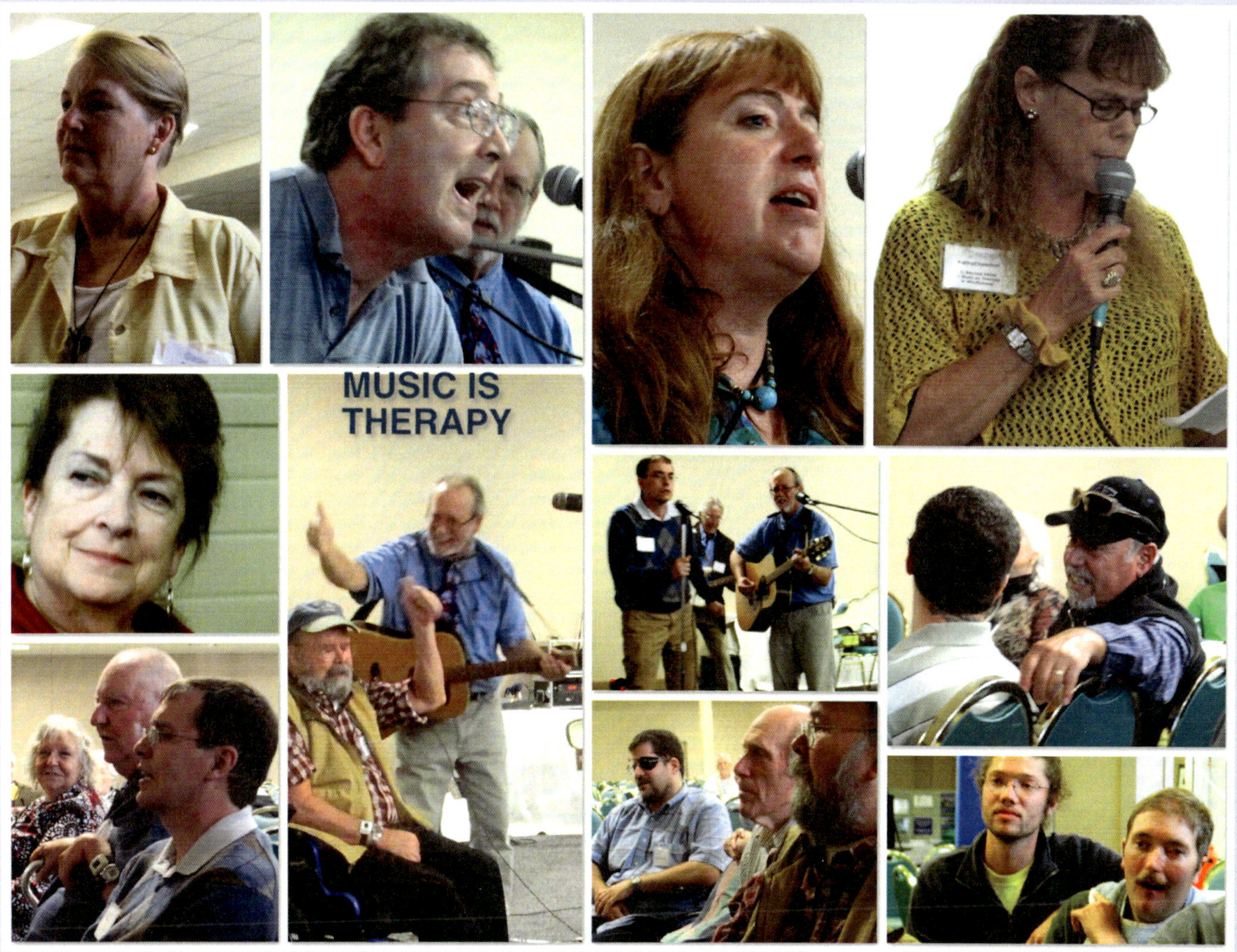

"Over time, I've realized it is true that we can't give the clients all they want with their lives, the exact life they had before their injury and sometimes you do wish you could do more, undo what happened. But what you can do is make their daily life as enjoyable as possible. That's what I try to remember every day."

—Butch Towsley

verse. It's a big step; just months ago, McLellan wasn't speaking at all.

"What do you want to sing next?" Miller-Wade, a lifelong musician who plays in several popular Grateful Dead cover bands, asks.

"Stewball!" the clients shout out, as Miller-Wade hands the guitar over to Kathy Chandler, who runs Emma's Place. This is her song and the clients love its simplicity and familiarity. It's a moment to behold, clients and staff grinning as they sing about a horse that is the underdog in a race but wins in the end.

The use of music in therapy for the brain has evolved rapidly in recent years as brain-imaging techniques have revealed the brain's plasticity—its ability to change—and have identified networks that music activates. Knowing this, doctors, researchers and therapists have increasingly used music to retrain the injured brain – just as Dr. William Frey did with Lenny Burke back in the early 1980s. Long before it became acceptable practice, Frey was using the popular Credence Clearwater Revival song "Proud Mary" to help Lenny remember basketball statistics and, in so doing, rebuild brain synapses.

How is it that people who have lost their ability to talk can sing and that song can stimulate improvements in motor control? The answers are complex and still being studied but researchers now know that singing, which relies mainly on right-hemisphere brain systems, can bypass injured left-hemisphere speech centers. More simply, singing comes from a different part of our brains than spoken language. It's as if singing opens a kind of back door to an undamaged part of the brain, a part that can be trained in some cases to take over the part that used to control speech. Indeed, Arizona Representative Gabrielle Giffords, who survived a gunshot wound to the left hemisphere of her brain, has used music therapy as a way of regaining her voice and ability to communicate.

Also, music tends to activate the brain bilaterally – both sides of the brain are engaged – and, while the evidence indicates that it's more of a right brain activity, it's also thought that music may create and activate neural responses throughout the brain and enhance the way the whole brain works. For example, researchers discovered that learning word lists in a song rather than just saying them activates temporal and frontal brain areas on both sides of the brain, while spoken-word learning activates areas only located in the brain's left hemisphere.

This research has been used in early child education from recordings like "School House Rock" or television shows like Sesame Street. Applying this knowledge to people with learning problems based on damage to a part of the brain only makes sense.

Researchers have also discovered recently that music activates what's called the "attention network" on both sides of the brain, meaning that music can be used to help people with strokes or brain injuries overcome attention problems. The implications of this for people with attention deficit disorder and similar conditions are exciting.

Now researchers are investigating whether music can also be used to reteach motor control to people with a host of conditions from traumatic brain injury to Parkinson's Disease. The reason lies within the brain itself, where music and motor control share circuits. Indeed, biomedical researchers have found that music is in itself a highly structured auditory language involving complex perception, cognition, and motor control in the brain, and thus it can effectively be used to retrain and reeducate the injured brain for a whole range of yet still unexplored recoveries.

And, so, at Lenny Burke's Farm, they sing. They sing with joy and hope.

Gary Miller-Wade

Gary Miller-Wade has only had one real mentor in his life, the man they call Rev at Lenny Burke's Farm. He's referring to the late-Rev. Richard Marceau, who was co-director of the farm from its early days until his death a few years ago. "He was just a good man," Miller-Wade says. "He had belief, but he didn't push it on you, religion, I mean. Amidst people who are troubled and in need, he had a way of calming everyone and making them feel like they were the best person they could be, or encourage them to strive to be the best person they could be.

"I try to keep it the way he ran it," Miller-Wade says, referring to the Thursday group sing-a-longs and discussion groups where residential clients, clients living in assisted apartments, individuals who have sustained traumatic brain injuries living in the wider community and staff gather for support and conversation.

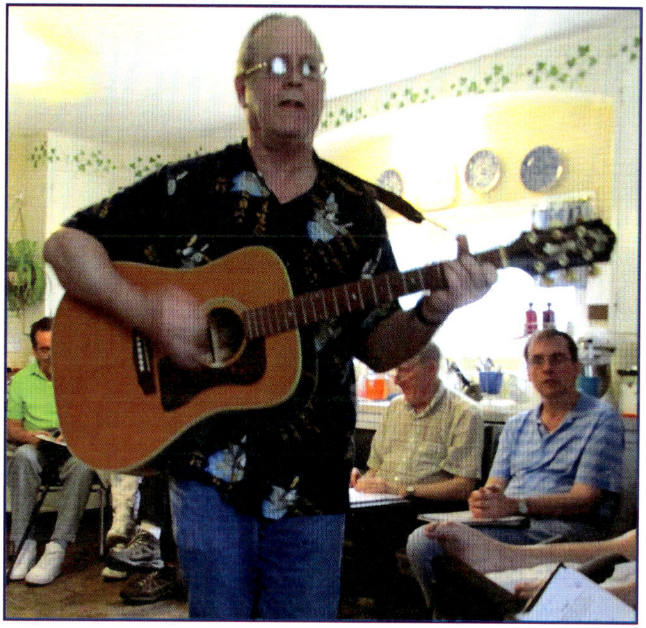

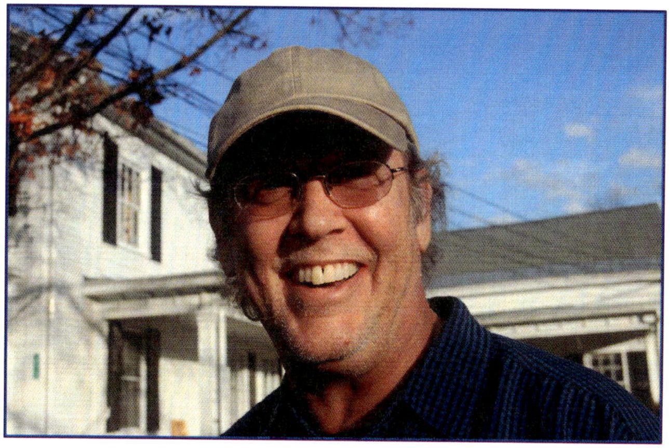

Music and helping people who have disabilities are integral for Miller-Wade, 61; the two pursuits have been constants in his life since an early age. A graduate of the Berklee College of Music, he has long played in several popular Grateful Dead tribute bands. Along with being the musical director at Lenny Burke's Farm, he serves as a one-on-one aide to a client who now lives on his own, Jean McDuff. Additionally, Miller-Wade and his wife Susan provide care for clients with disabilities who live with them in their home.

Like just about everyone who has been at the farm since the days when Rev led the Thursday groups, Miller-Wade misses him "every day. He was perfect for where he was meant to be," Miller-Wade says. Indeed, it was the spirit that he felt when he first met Rev and watched him in action that's kept him working at the farm for eight years.

And one gets the feeling, watching Miller-Wade as he plays his guitar and sings with the clients, smiling and encouraging and accepting, that he, too, is where he was meant to be.

talking out of need but out of desire, as in asking for chocolate chip ice cream, a request that quite convinced Upton that Lenny's brain was functioning at a level beyond his understanding. Soon, Upton was sharing the ice cream request with the hospital staff.

Word got to David Wolk and Jack Healey who were on the radio working the second day of the fundraiser; they made the announcement that Lenny had spoken his first words and that among them was a request for ice cream. Almost immediately, people were cheering in the streets of Rutland. Within hours of the news that Lenny had asked for chocolate chip ice cream, the hospital's freezers were overflowing with his favorite flavor. At Mass the next day, Father Richard Lavalley knew how to get a standing ovation. He told the congregation that Lenny was talking and the congregation stood up and clapped, something that was certainly not done in Catholic churches in 1979.

"To me, that was so magical," David Wolk recalls. "Here's the entire community coming together to support Lenny and his family. Jack Healey's talking about Lenny on the radio and he hears that and wakes up."

Lenny had woken up on March 9. The next day he made it clear he knew that March 10 was Kevin's birthday. When he wasn't talking, he was praying that Kevin would not get his driver's license, that he'd fail the driver's test. That day and for some time into the future, whenever the subject of his brain injury came up, Lenny refused to believe it had occurred on a basketball court. Perhaps he'd been in a car accident, or a bicycle accident, or fallen and hit his head. Kevin should not get his license; he might get injured as badly as Lenny had.

This was just one of his obsessions as he awoke and, as he began to talk, it became clear that Lenny, as his mother suspected, had been aware of what was going on around him all through his weeks of unconsciousness. He knew, for example, that he had missed Kathy's birthday on February 20 and was full of apologies about that, even expressing the sentiment that he understood that his injuries had wrecked her birthday. He knew he had had a date the night after his injury and was angry to have missed it. He asked his mother how old he was because the things she had praised during the night when he was in such critical condition were mostly from when he was younger. Why hadn't she mentioned his early acceptance to college?

One of the more humorous conversations that is told about Lenny's first days out of the coma was one he had with Dr. Upton. "Thank you for saving my life," he told the doctor who of course, responded, "You're welcome," whereupon Lenny is said to have quipped, "Well, don't think you did it all alone."

Lenny also said he had heard Upton tell his parents he might die. How did he know all these things? How had he kept track of time while in a coma? Emmie will tell you it was because he was always there, present, even at the worst moments. She believes it was also because of Jim Kelley. Lenny had memorized the schedule for the basketball season, what night his team was playing which school. He knew the strengths and weaknesses of the opposing team members, many of whom he had played in previous seasons. As Kelley came to the hospital every night, he would ask Lenny what he should do to prepare for the next game. "So, Lenny we're going to play ...," the coach would say. "You know how strong they are on defense. What strategy would you suggest?" Then he would come in after a game and go through the game, play by play, telling Lenny how it had gone down, what had worked and what had not.

Emmie believes that these conversations more than anything else kept her son grounded in time. "Jim was building synapses all through Lenny's stay at the hospital. It wasn't just a one-way street. Jim had come to MSJ in Lenny's freshman year; he had never coached a game there without Lenny so it was essential for him to go over the plays with Lenny as well."

As Emmie later realized, Lenny's brain was already exercising its neuroplasticity – the brain's ability to reorganize itself by forming new neural connections – and it was his coach and mentor, Jim Kelley, among others, who was helping him. Lenny tells us, however, that at the same time, like Emmie, he might well have been somewhere between living and dying. Indeed, as he later told a reporter, "In the hospital, I could hear things that people said when I was unconscious. The people were careful not to say too much or speak too loudly, even though I wasn't supposed to be able to hear. In fact, during the time that I was in a coma, I often felt that I was in heaven with God. I can remember it exactly – it was light blue all around. I love God. I know he pulled me through. I was in both places at once, here on earth and also in heaven."

It's hard to imagine how Emmie, her husband Len and the other children, the players and all those who had sat around Lenny's hospital room, or gathered at the Burkes' house, all those who had followed the news of his struggle with death for a month and a half, felt upon hearing that Lenny had not just awoken but spoken sentences that made sense. Indeed, with the pressure removed from his head, Lenny began to speak a lot, sometimes nonstop and certainly much more garrulously than he had before the injury.

The difference was noticeable. Even Lenny knew it. After he had talked for 56 hours straight, exhausting everyone to the point that they might wish he would just shut up, Lenny made everyone laugh by saying, "You know I'm talking more like Kevin now," referring to his more gregarious brother. Even today he likes to joke about how he went from a shy, quiet fellow to an extroverted one.

Once it was clear that the shunt had stabilized the pressure in Lenny's brain and that he was not going to die, he was transferred from the Rutland Hospital to the DeGoesbriand unit of the Burlington Medical Center where, on April 2, he started physical therapy under the care of Richard Nixon's cousin, Dr. Raymond Milhous, a physiatrist. Emmie stayed nearby and spent quite a bit of time with Lenny, attending his physical therapy sessions – not just as mom, but also as student. She was learning as much as possible. She knew that the journey to recovery would be long and she wanted as many tools as possible.

Kathy, being 11 at the time, was around much of the time. She was still young enough that she loved playing teacher with Lenny whenever she visited him, their roles of youngest and oldest almost reversed. Happily, the two would play word games for hours. However, Kathy was quite bothered that during his unconsciousness Lenny's face had sagged on the left side, an effect of the head injury similar to what happens to some people who sustain strokes. She was sure she could get Lenny's old smile back. Like her mother, going on instinct and hope, Kathy thought Lenny just had to remember how to smile and frown and then these natural, autonomic movements would come back. She would help him remember by rebuilding his facial muscles. She devised a game wherein she would push his face up into a smile or down into a frown and time how long Lenny could hold the pose. In one variation of the game, she'd cover his face with a facecloth then tell him to smile or frown, then take the cloth away. Over

Christopher Patrick Russell: There Are Only Good Memories There

Sometimes, it simply makes no sense.

Christopher Patrick Russell was probably driving from visiting one girlfriend to see another, sober and carefree one moment, fighting for his life the next. His mother, Leslie Kittell-Emerson of Sheldon, Vermont, says he liked to have several girlfriends at a time, each in a different town so they might not run into one another.

"He used to say to me, 'I'm young. I like to play the field.' Everyone loved him; he's that kind of person, a real sweetheart."

Russell's work shift had ended the previous day at 3 a.m. and, since he had the next day off, rather than go home to bed, he'd spent the night driving from Colchester where he worked to visit various friends in northern Vermont. A group of them were following in their own car when Russell suddenly crossed the road and plowed under an SUV. Remarkably, he survived the crash with what appeared to be simply a broken right wrist and left leg.

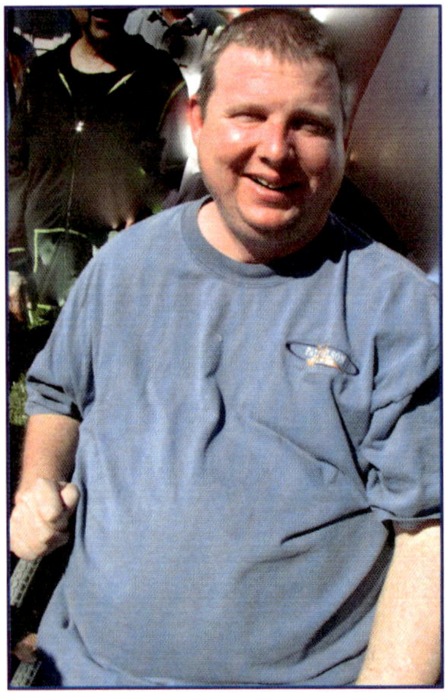

Kittell-Emerson says police found a six-pack on the backseat but no alcohol in Russell. And even though it was winter, just a few days before Christmas when the accident occurred, the roads weren't slippery. Most likely, Russell had fallen asleep. He was 21 years old.

At the emergency room in Burlington, something went wrong as the doctors were setting his broken bones. They had discovered a large blood clot in his neck, stopped the surgery and found themselves working to simply keep him alive. He died three times that night.

Somehow he was stabilized but he was in a coma for months, during which he either had a stroke or part of the blood clot went to his brain, and that – and not the car accident per se – caused paralysis and brain damage, resulting in some short-term memory loss and communication problems.

"It's been very hard," Kittell-Emerson says. "We are very close. He looks like me, acts like me; we have the same disposition. We even like the same music – Jimi Hendrix, Led Zeppelin, all that."

She describes a son who was confident, popular, funny and self-reliant. For example, one night, not wanting to stay over at a friend's house nor wake the friend, Russell walked several miles home in freezing weather, wearing only a T-shirt and jeans. He was generous with his time, she recalls, helping farm neighbors in season. "He was very strong, not big like now, just strong. He could throw two 200-pound hay bales at once."

The trail to Lenny Burke's Farm took Russell from Mary Fletcher Hospital in Burlington, now the Fletcher Allen Medical Center, to the old DeGoesbriand Hospital, then Crotched Mountain in New Hampshire.

At Emma's Place, Russell likes to sit on the porch facing the town's main street, listen to music and comment on the women and cars as they pass by. He waves and says hello to anyone he sees, cheerfully. As his mother says, "He always was a happy kid."

He's 39 now. His vocabulary is sparse; his mobility as well, but he is working hard with therapists to improve his flexibility. He smiles often and sweetly. He excels at chess, checkers, cards; he's very mathematical. He rarely loses at the first two, occasionally on the third.

"It's hard to look at him now," Kittell-Emerson concedes. "I used to bring him home for visits but you drive into the St. Albans area, Fairfax, and his eyes tear up. He knows what he had. He's very happy at Emma's Place. There are only good memories there."

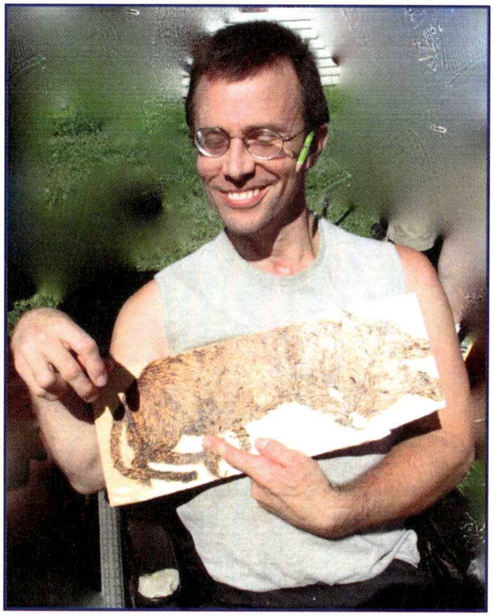

Jason O'Connor and his cat. He created this picture with his wood-burning tool.

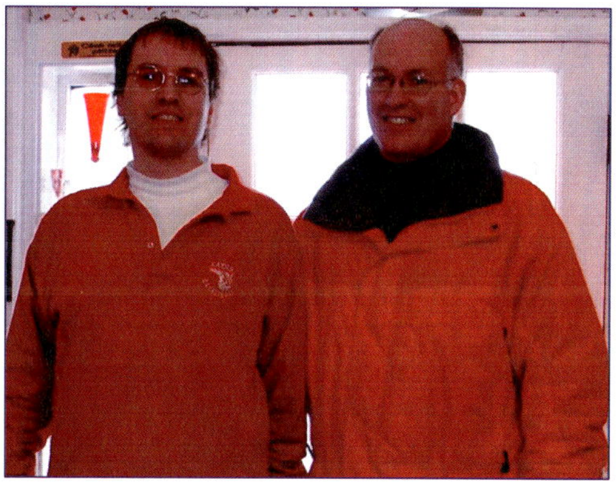

Lenny Burke and Randy Tabor, a childhood friend who rarely left Lenny's side during his recovery.

Lenny's National Influence

By Dr. Ron Savage

Since Lenny's traumatic brain injury, much has changed in brain injury rehabilitation in this country. For me to be part of many of those changes has been an extraordinary adventure, but I also know that without Lenny being my "Ground Zero," I would never have had such an interesting career. You will see below that I "blame" many things on Lenny over the years because these are all threads that lead back to his influence upon me.

While we had special education services for students starting in the mid-1970s, we had never included students, like Lenny, with "traumatic brain injury" (TBI). Students with TBI were not well understood and were often classified as students with some other type of learning disability. (This is like a physician diagnosing someone with the wrong disease and then prescribing the wrong medicine.) In the late 1980s I started working with the late Senator Robert Stafford, a Republican from Vermont, and his staff to include TBI as a special education classification in the Individuals with Disabilities Education Act (IDEA). Thanks to Senator Stafford, hearings were held, meeting set up, and in 1991 TBI became part of our national special education laws. This is now law in every state and all the "Lennys" with TBI are now being properly identified and receiving the services and supports they need in school and college.

Teacher training was also an issue for students with TBI. Identifying students with TBI was important, but understanding TBI and how to best help the student was not a part of any teacher training programs. While I was a professor at Castleton State College, I was allowed time in my schedule (1984) to create the first-ever manual for teachers, An Educator's Manual: What teachers need to know about students with traumatic brain injuries.

My colleagues who worked with me also had "Lenny-like" experiences and we collated our knowledge to help teachers and therapists better understand TBI in children and adolescents. This manual later became a textbook, Educational Dimensions of Acquired Brain Injury (1995). At the same time in the early 1990s, we also created the first master's program in TBI at George Washington University and, more recently, an on-line training certificate program for teachers. Since teachers were not the only ones craving education about TBI, in 1994, as a founding member working with others, I helped establish the Academy for the Certification of Brain Injury Specialists (ACBIS) and have now provided training to well over 2,500 professionals in the United States.

Lastly, when Emmie and I first went looking for information on TBI, not only did we find very little, but most of it was in medical textbooks and articles that did not help families with the day-to-day, long term struggles that people face. In 1996, with three other colleagues, we established LA Publishing, which produces materials for families, teachers, therapists, psychologists, and others who are working day-to-day with individuals with brain injuries. This is now the largest publishing company of its kind and, once again, these are all threads that can be traced back to Lenny.

Working with Emmie over the years, her words have always echoed in my head, "This is not just about Lenny. There are hundreds of other Vermonters in the same situation." Not only that, there are millions of survivors of TBI in the United States. The Centers for Disease Control and prevention report that every year at least 3.5 million Americans experience a traumatic brain injury, which is a leading cause of injury, death and disability in the United States that affects persons of all ages, races/ethnicities and incomes. As I learned with Emmie and Lenny, professional knowledge about people with TBI is critical.

As chairman of the North American Brain Injury Society (NABIS) that educates professionals about TBI, and editor of our journal, Brain Injury Professional, I know from those early days in Vermont that the more we know the better we will deliver ("translating brain injury science into practice.") As I look back, there was certainly no crystal ball to tell us how far Lenny would heal, but unless we stepped up as professionals we would never find out. So many times Lenny has amazed me and his gains have inspired me to keep pushing for new and better services for people with TBI, especially young people. I also chair the International Pediatric Brain Injury Society, which has members around the world. It was not just about Lenny, or Vermonters, or US citizens, TBI is a world-wide issue.

Even today, as we look at the nearly 1 million young men and women returning from wars in Iraq and Afghanistan, TBI has become the "signature wound" of these wars because of blasts and IEDs. Our Veterans Administration hospitals are being overwhelmed with this population of survivors and the complexity of TBI. Sadly, the average age of these young veterans is 19.3 years, not much older than Lenny when he was injured. While we have made great strides in brain injury rehabilitation, we are still a long ways from preventing, identifying, and treating TBI.

Emmie, Lenny and I used to travel to Washington, DC, for the National Head Injury Foundation with other families to try and influence Congress to provide more support for people with TBI and their families. Our Vermont representatives were always helpful, especially Senators Stafford and Leahy. The key to our success was that "Everyone knew Lenny." Lenny's story had become so well known that we had no problems explaining what TBI was and/or the kinds of supports people like Lenny needed. Lenny has become an ambassador for TBI. When Lenny spoke, everyone listened.

While I could talk about Lenny's TBI and the needs of individuals with TBI for hours, it was Lenny who provided the most riveting testimony. To this day whenever I am working in Washington, DC, I always have a parent or person with a TBI with me. Nothing is more powerful. Lenny taught me that.

Fortunately, since Lenny's injury, Congress has addressed many issues related to brain policies and funding, primarily with the Departments of Education (ED) and Health and Human Services (HHS) and more recently within the Departments of Defense and Veterans Affairs for research, treatment, rehabilitation and care for veterans and returning service members with TBI and their families. These achievements include:

- Since 1987, appropriations to the National Institute on Disability Rehabilitation and Research (NIDRR) for TBI Model Systems (16 centers) and the TBI Model Systems National Data Center;
- NIDRR currently funding two Rehabilitation Research & Training Centers on TBI and associated research projects. The two currently funded RR&T Centers are: Developing Strategies to Foster Community Integration and Participation (TIRR Memorial Hermann and Baylor College of Medicine in Houston, TX) and Center on Interventions for Children and Youth (Children's Medical Center, Cincinnati, OH);
- The 1990 Individuals with Disabilities Education Act reauthorization added TBI as a disability category;
- The TBI Act of 1996, as amended, authorizing funding to:
    - The Centers for Disease Control and Prevention (CDC) to determine incidence and prevalence of TBI, conduct public awareness and prevention programs;
    - The National Institutes of Health (NIH) to conduct TBI research; and
    - The Health Resources and Services Administration (HRSA) for state grants to improve service delivery. The 2000 amendments authorized funding to HRSA to expand advocacy services provided by state Protection & Advocacy Systems to include individuals with TBI; and
- Enactment of the Dignified Treatment of Wounded Warriors Act as part of the National Defense Authorization Act of 2008, the landmark legislation establishing the Defense Centers of Excellence for TBI and Psychological Health, mandating pre- and post-deployment screening of service members, extending coverage periods for military insurance beneficiaries and authorizing the U.S. Department of Veterans Affairs to contract with civilian providers for hospital care and medical services.
- The Patient Protection and Affordable Care Act, which defined essential health care benefits to include rehabilitation and provides incentives to states to improve long-term services and supports to individuals with disabilities and older adults.

- Funding for the Project B.R.A.I.N. initiative ($100 M), which is the Brain Research through Advancing Innovative Neurotechnologies (BRAIN) Initiative aimed at revolutionizing our understanding of the human brain in order to help people suffering from such devastating conditions as TBI.

Most recently, I was involved in educating and helping states pass Youth Sports Concussion Laws across the country. Fourty-nine states, including Vermont, have passed Sports Concussions laws that aim to (1) require schools to baseline test their student-athletes before the season starts, (2) to screen and monitor concussions in student-athletes, and (3) to make sure no athlete returns to play until symptom free and cleared by a medical professional. When I think of Lenny sustaining a severe TBI in a basketball game, I also think of the millions of young people each year who sustain concussions and more severe brain injuries on our athletic fields and recreational parks. Even the NFL has recognized its role in the management of concussions and the long term effects that brain injuries have on its players.

Looking back on my time with Lenny and all that I learned from him, I am so appreciative of being one of many people in his life whom he has profoundly impacted in a positive way. Besides my sons, there is no other individual who has influenced me more as a person or as a professional. Working with Lenny was an honor I will never forget. Having him now as a friend is as good as life gets.

An estimated 1.6 million to 3.8 million sports-related TBIs occur each year.

Daniel Patrick Fanning: Peace and Love and Hope in Yourself

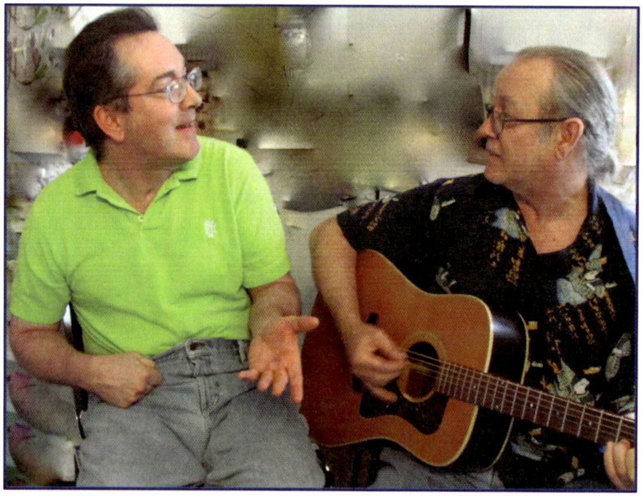

Daniel Patrick Fanning singing "Danny Boy," with Gary Miller-Wade, who leads the weekly group meetings.

People call Danny Fanning, 52, a hero; he saved his wife and children's lives but sustained a horrible head injury when another vehicle slammed into the car he was driving on Mother's Day, 1990. Fanning took the brunt of the hit, turning the driver's side of his vehicle into the collision to absorb the impact just seconds after he realized there was no escaping it.

Fanning barely survived. Besides a broken jaw, he was in a deep coma for weeks and when he awoke he had great difficulty walking and was very confused, almost incommunicative. He spent almost two months in the hospital, then the Sargent Rehabilitation Center at Newport Hospital in Rhode Island, then another rehab center in Virginia. Finally, when the therapists said there was nothing more they could do, the Fannings took their son home, where he lived for a year and a half.

"You never saw anyone who liked to work like Danny did. He loved his family. Now he had to accept the fact that he had to be cautious, that he had to learn how to walk all over again and use a cane. He had to come to terms with the fact that his wife couldn't take care of him, the boys and work. We did our best but we were just collapsing" from caring for him, Fanning's father Dan says.

At first the Fannings were both guilt-ridden and broken-hearted to leave their son at Lenny Burke's Farm. "When we first left him here and after our first visits, as we drove away we would begin to weep," Dan Fanning says.

"If you knew Danny before the accident and saw him then …," he says, his voice heavy with memory and loss. "But eventually, we saw how well he was doing here and we stopped weeping."

As his father's voice trails off, Danny Fanning senses the sadness in the room. Getting awkwardly to his feet, he fills the quiet with the words he's most apt to say, a personal mantra that he repeats often each day.

"Peace," he says, smiling at his parents and giving them the peace sign. "Harmony. And love. And hope. Hope in yourself and hope in the world."

These are also the words that are repeated at the end of each week's group session and sing-along where, undoubtedly, Fanning will have requested his favorite song, "Danny Boy."

He knows all the words.

At least 5.3 million Americans, 2 percent of the U.S. population, currently live with disabilities resulting from TBI.

The Case of Lenny B

By William F. Frey, Ph.D.
Retired Psychotherapist and educator,
Middlebury College and Castleton College

Throughout my clinical training, case studies often provided that insightful, subjective reality that poorly proven theories overlooked. It has become apparent over the years of working as a therapist that clinicians often learn so much more from their patient than they are able to give back. I felt this way with Lenny B.

Lenny was referred to me because I had training in behavioral therapies (the application of learning principles to psychological problems) and neuropsychology (the budding specialty that measured and described brain–behavior relationships). At the time of his injury and treatment, the prevailing wisdom limited psychotherapy to only those patients who appeared to have "intact" brains. Fortunately, I had no such prejudice.

Lenny had a smile that required reciprocation and a glint in his eyes that said, "I am aware, intelligent and ready to learn." His gait was strange for a young man and his fine motor movements limited, but he had retained the grace of an athlete. He conversed enthusiastically about all subjects without self-monitoring or censor. He was constantly exploring every aspect of my office while asking question after question about my life and interests. I learned quickly that a therapeutic bond was easily established, although he seemed to remember little of previous sessions except for my name and those of my staff. Today, his symptoms are considered variations of classic traumatic brain injury (TBI) sequelae, but at the time were simply clinically fascinating.

Lenny provided early and significant evidence that, regardless of the type or severity of a traumatic brain injury, a client can maintain attachments and establish a therapeutic bond.

Therapy with adolescents or young adults living at home requires a family systems evaluation; interventions that considered the family dynamic were critical to success. Interviews with his mother and father suggested an underlying chaos expected after the seriousness of Lenny's accident, but the push for equilibrium was coming from his mother and seemed fueled by more than just acceptance of his injury.

It was apparent that having his mother, Emmie, in sessions was critical. Details related to Lenny's current symptom expressions, basic daily activity reports, progress with prescribed exercises and emotional wellbeing could be reliably tracked with her help. In addition, she could provide explanations of his behavior and discuss these in relation to past personality features and current variants. The sessions also seemed to provide support for Emmie. Although I hadn't realized the significance, this would be a model for most of my future work with TBI patients.

As Emmie became more versed in the medical model and Lenny's care, her personal goals focused on more education, understanding and rehabilitation systems. Her constant quest for support services, treatment direction, academic support and family health kept everyone she contacted questioning what we could devise to help. In this regard, not only the medical community but also the entire Rutland community worked to help and track Lenny's progress. He had been a small town hero, hurt doing what should have just been fun, and everyone empathized and rallied to make it as right as such a situation could be. It seemed as though everyone knew it could be their son or daughter, which made Lenny's condition personal.

Memory is critical to cognitive functioning. A therapy that just relied on talking would be limited to the session if the patient couldn't recall what was talked about. Having a third party such as Emmie relate what we discussed was helpful, but it was thought that including another person in the session might skew the topics/emotions discussed and break the therapeutic alliance and trust between patient and therapist. Fortunately, Lenny demonstrated that there were many types of memory and that strategies can be developed to improve performance so that sessions were not wasted.

Two examples remain vivid for me. Early in our sessions, Lenny discovered a blue and white apothecary jar in my office that had candies in it. Almost each subsequent session he seemed to discover it again and as always would have a piece of candy. One session the jar had coincidently been removed. Lenny came in, sat down, looked at me and said, "Dr. Frey, where is the candy jar?" This seemed monumental to me then, embarrassing now, but so instructive as an example of how memory and learning operate. Repetition and reward became the treatment model for the next months with slow but steady gains.

On another occasion, Emmie was relating to me that she and Lenny had been to Burlington for a doctor's appointment and that the trip was fine for Lenny, as he had sung songs along with the radio the whole way up. I off-handedly asked how he knew the words, was it an oldies station. She looked at me quizzically and said, no these were new songs. I kept a guitar in my office for practice and to use in some clinical situations, so I tried a few examples with Lenny and found that he could recall information that had a musical melody. We used the NCAA basketball pairings as an example and he was able to sing 32 pairings to the Credence Clearwater Revival song "Proud Mary" melody. This provided a hopeful clue that cognitive functioning can be improved and that music could be used as a tool in the treatment of people with TBI.

Because of the TBI, Lenny needed to relearn some social skills. In this, I relied on the current research on assertiveness training with recognition of facial expressions and body language being highlighted. It seemed that individuals who could not pick up on facial expressions or body language or were too attentive to them had difficulty in social interactions. Practicing those skills helped reduce the uncomfortable situations Lenny would find himself in as he began to read people's feedback more efficiently. Again, much repetition and practice were required but, as he regained many of these skills, he provided another example or way of understanding neuroplasticity, the ability of the brain to relearn and change throughout life.

Guidelines for behavioral therapists in the 1980s in regard to the relationship between the patient and the therapist were murky. For example, therapists would work on phobia issues in real life situations, such as taking a patient to a store or riding an elevator with them, literally being with the patient in the situation that provided the difficulty. This was a new behavioral model.

I would hear Emmie talk about how difficult it was at times at home with his siblings and in everyday situations. I could not seem to understand in a way that was helpful. It occurred to me that if Lenny could spend a weekend with my family, maybe I would have a better understanding of what she meant. But in doing so I was stretching the proscribed boundaries in that I would be bringing a client into my home for observation and interaction.

I rationalize this boundary stretch 30 years later as Lenny was just wonderful with my very young children and my wife. (Today, he still remembers their names and asks about them.) Through the experience, I realized the subtly overpowering level of responsibility it is to care for someone with cognitive and physical needs. The needs for home support and rehabilitation that are considered standard now became so clear to me after that weekend and I could never again take for granted the challenges a family faces dealing with these issues.

There are fortunate coincidences that occur in one's career. One night while at a social gathering at a friend's home, one of my friends shared she had these strange symptoms that none of her doctors seemed to understand. She described her symptoms of the past three months, headaches, tiredness, forgetting and focus. Her doctors thought she should see a therapist as they sounded like "It was all in her head." Her symptoms reminded me of Lenny's and other TBI patients I was now treating, so I inquired as to when they began. She said she was working in the barn when she somehow hit her head. I began to investigate some of the models proposed to explain what were considered "minor" brain trauma and it was clear that her injuries were the result of a concussion. With some reassurance and time my friend recovered and I learned that every brain injury is significant. Had I not treated Lenny I might never have put the obvious connection between concussive injuries and traumatic brain injuries together.

My investigation into the spectrum of brain trauma, its consequences, and rehabilitation spanned my entire career as a psychotherapist and as an educator at Middlebury College and Castleton College. My early experiences with Lenny's treatment gave me hope for every patient I would see. More importantly, science has provided data to support so many of our early efforts with Lenny and no one could have predicted the rehabilitation universe Emmie and other parents like her would create that

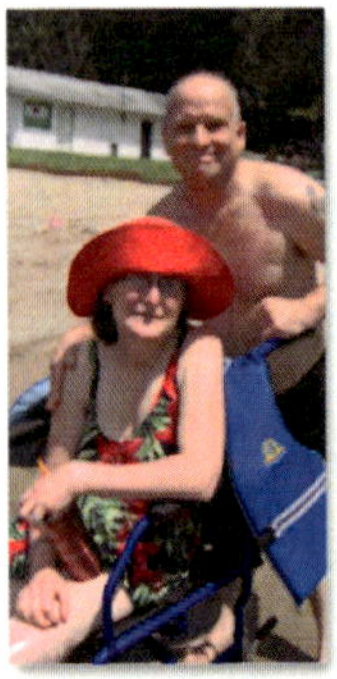

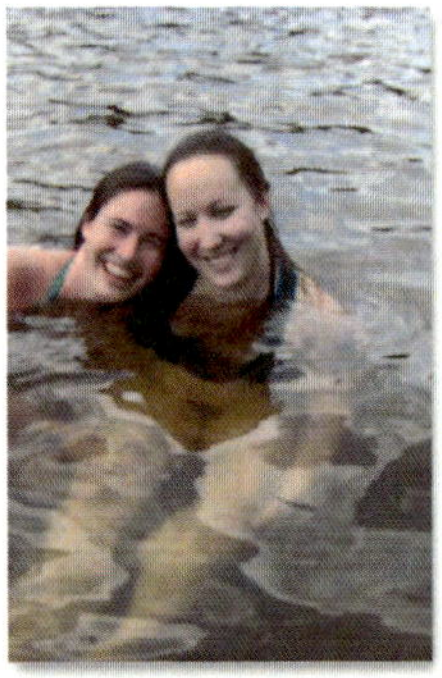

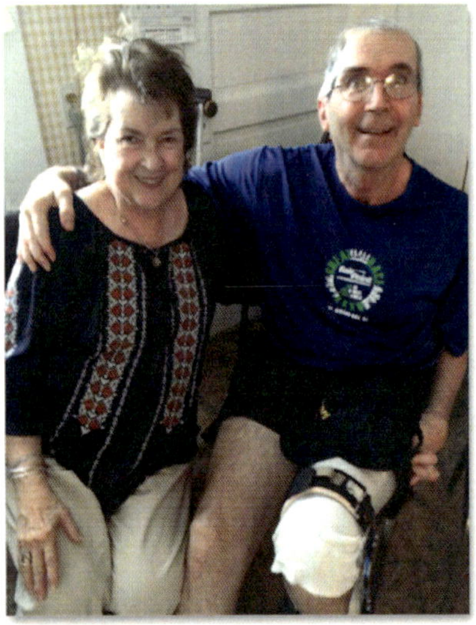

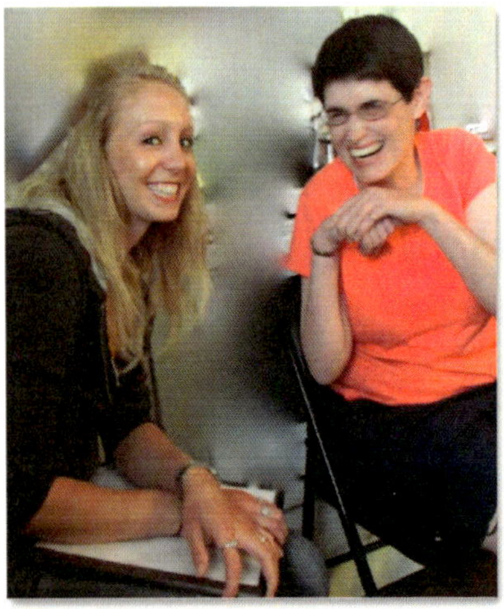

revolutionized rehabilitation medicine. It will not surprise me that the treatment models developed for Lenny and other patients with brain injury will become the norm for all psychotherapy patients regardless of diagnosis. Understanding there is no value in the "intact" brain model but rather understanding brains are constantly evolving, unique to each of us, and very trainable was the lesson Lenny taught us all. There are so many brave patients with all kinds of illnesses and conditions that guide us professionals toward questions and answers we would never have broached had we not treated them. Thank you Lenny, Emmie and family for including me.

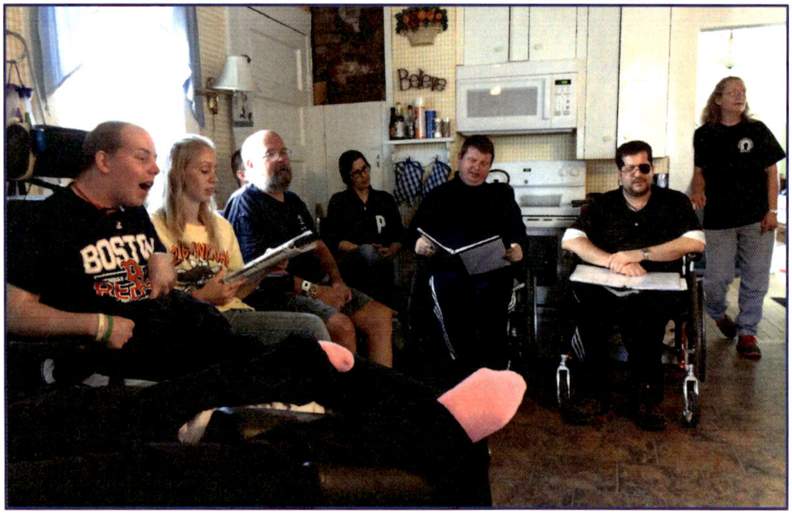

The new kid at Lenny Burke's Farm, Christopher Christian, left, joins other clients and staff members Kayla Werner, George Parton, Kendra Bowman, Christopher Patrick Russell, Rich Martineit and Lynne Keyes at the Thursday Sing-a-long at Emma's Place.

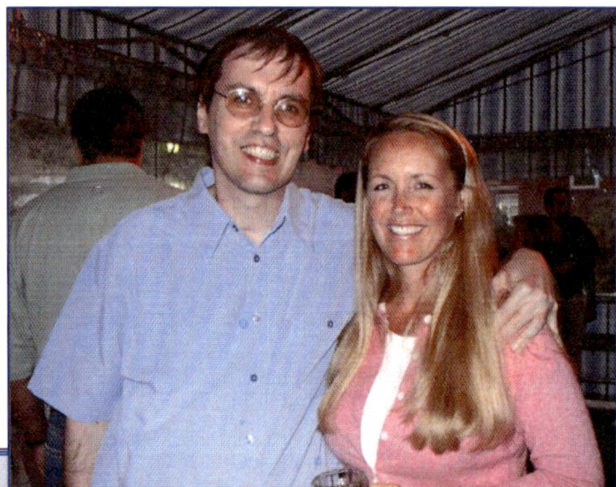

Lenny Burke and Lisa Sullivan Shappy at their 25th class reunion!

BTF
BRAIN TRAUMA FOUNDATION

CDC
CENTERS FOR DISEASE CONTROL AND PREVENTION

A-Head Check

IMMEDIATE HEAD INJURY EVALUATION

Alert

Is the person alert? Question him/her:

- Can you open your eyes?
- Can you explain to me what happened?

If there is no response to either question immediately call 911 for medical assistance.

Ask

If the person is alert, ask him/her:

- Do you have a severe headache?
- Do you feel like you may vomit?
- Do you have difficulty staying awake?

If the answer is yes to any of these questions or if the person has any symptoms that concern you, seek medical assistance or call 911.

Aid

All head injuries should be evaluated by an appropriate healthcare professional. A hit on the head can cause a brain injury.

- Brain injuries can range from mild (mild concussion) to severe (coma)
- Symptoms may appear hours or days later

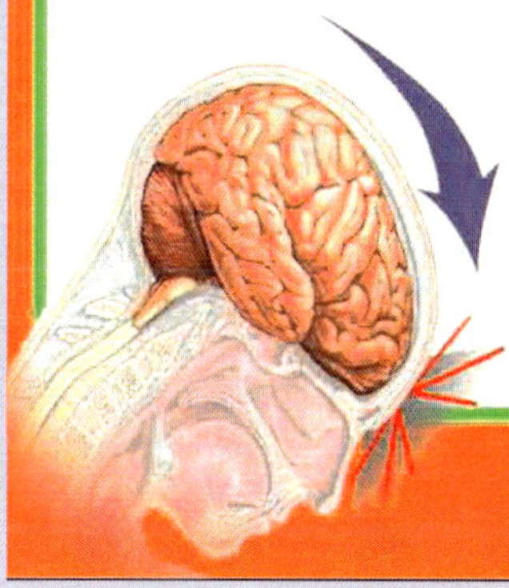

After a brain injury, the person should rest and not engage in any activities requiring a lot of concentration or physical activity until symptom free.

For more information, visit **www.braintrauma.org** or **www.cdc.gov/Concussion.**

A part of CDC's Heads Up Series

Every year, approximately 52,000 deaths occur from traumatic brain injury.

time, the muscles got stronger and Lenny regained the ability to control his facial muscles. Indeed, as she had guessed, Kathy had helped Lenny rebuild not just the muscles of the face but the brain synapsis that controlled them.

Lenny's first visit home was on Easter, April 15, 1979. His return, however, was bittersweet because as happy as Lenny was to be home, and as happy as everyone was to have him home, Lenny more deeply realized his limitations. When last in this house, he had been the basketball champ, the oldest brother making college plans and dreaming of life after high school, the kid with the driver's license. Now, his eye was quite deviated, limiting his ability to see. Having been hospitalized for so long, his muscles had atrophied and he was weak; his left side was semi-paralyzed and, although he could stand, he couldn't get to his feet on his own or support his weight for any amount of time. And it was his younger brother who now asked for the keys to his mother's car.

Nonetheless, his siblings being still children wanted to know if Lenny could still shoot hoops. One day, they took him outside and stood him in front of the basketball hoop. Despite the vision and strength issues and the lack of coordination, Lenny just kept making one basket after another. They thought it was a miracle. Later, therapists explained how Lenny was able to do this. He was operating from deep-seated memory, not from sight. The memory of shooting baskets was deeply imbedded in his muscles and brain from years and years of practice.

Long-term memory, of course, was far different from short term; Lenny's brain injury had most dramatically affected his short-term memory. His short-term memory wasn't completely annihilated. He could remember some things that had recently occurred while other events, with no particular rhyme or reason, remained irretrievable. Further complicating communication was the fact that Lenny could remember things that he had heard while he was still in his coma but might forgot something he had been told repeatedly after he regained consciousness.

For example, his cousin Chris Vignoe had told Lenny about the day Chris and his friends had needed $10 for pizza while they were hanging out at the Burke house, tired of eating the endless casseroles that friends and relatives dropped off. Anyone who knew Lenny knew that he liked money, was very good at saving it and always knew precisely how much he had at any given time and in what denomination. While Lenny was still in his coma, Chris confided to Lenny that he had borrowed $10 from his bedroom drawer for the pizza, but paid it back, not to worry. One of the first things Lenny wanted to do when he got home was "see what those kids have done with my money."

His room was upstairs but the kid who always took two or three steps at a time couldn't climb stairs. He needed Kevin and Emmie, pushing and pulling from either end, to help him. When he got to his room, he went right to his drawer. The amount was right, but not in the denominations that he had put there all those months ago. And Lenny knew that.

At the same time, every time Emmie's mother Dorothy visited, Lenny would be quite excited to see her but when she left he would ask why his other grandmother, Len's mother, never came to see him. Each time he was reminded that Grandma Burke had died – she had died six months previous to the day of Lenny's injuries in the same bed in the intensive care unit where Lenny had spent all those weeks – and each time Lenny was told she was dead he would be inconsolable as if hearing the news for the first time.

But then one day shortly into his recovery, he suddenly told his mother, "Oh, now I know why I thought Grandma Burke was alive. It was because I was in heaven with her. We spent a lot of time together there. That's why I miss her so much. I met your father there, too. He is so popular in heaven. He's so proud of his long white hair. We talked a lot but mostly I watched Obby play cards with his friends. He's quite the character, Mom."

It was the use of that nickname – Obby – that convinced Emmie that her son had indeed and inexplicably been with her father, whose name was Oliver James Ormsbee. His friends called him Obby. Because he was rather old when Emmie was born and had died when Emmie was just 11, she had few memories of him and barely knew the nickname herself. Indeed, with so colorful a mother, her stories rarely included much about her father, other than his early death. Besides, Lenny was the least interested of her children in family stories. Michael was the one who was fascinated with family history. She was sure that Lenny had never heard her father's nickname, as she never used it. And that business about his hair and his friends, what was that about? When she shared the story with her own mother, Dorothy confirmed that her father loved his hair and wore it rather long for the times and that he was a person who loved to socialize, play cards, and make new friends. And, indeed, he had been, as Lenny put it, quite a character.

"Rev would tell me Lenny is not entirely aware of being back. He's had this experience none of us have had. He's still a little bit in both places," Emmie says.

After progressing steadily in his physical therapy at the Burlington Medical Center, Lenny was allowed to move home on May 4, one hundred days after his injury. Three days later, Lenny made another major breakthrough – he walked using his own power for the first time since the injury. He was weak and a bit uncoordinated and the effort exhausted him after so much time in bed or a wheelchair, but he had walked. "I'll never forget the day he took his first steps," says Kathy. "Our family stood in a circle in our front yard as Lenny slowly and very unsteadily walked from one of us to the other."

At first he needed assistance with walking but, over a period of weeks, he became steadier and steadier and gained added confidence. Because walking was difficult, however, it took Lenny a while before he was doing it as voluntarily as he should, relying when he could on his wheelchair. Kevin had the notion that Lenny would never walk consistently on his own as long as he had the wheelchair to depend on. So, one day it just disappeared. (Of course it was handy if really needed but Kevin, like Emmie, knew that Lenny would not want to just sit around if the wheelchair were gone; he'd want to be where the action was. They hid it in the garage.)

Around the same time, Emmie also got rid of the hospital bed that took up much of the living room, not giving Lenny much privacy. Knowing that he wanted to sleep in his own bed, she came up with the idea of putting a twin-size mattress next to Lenny's bed upstairs where she would sleep and monitor his movement if he got up during the night. Eventually, she came to trust that he wouldn't fall out of the bed or try to go downstairs on his own and moved back to her own room.

Nonetheless, the next few weeks – and then the months ahead – proved to be some of the most demanding as hope and reality collided again and again. Despite the joy everyone felt with what they considered an almost miraculous awakening, especially on a day when the whole community

Brian Cavanaugh: Serendipity, Buddhism, Work and a Woman's Love

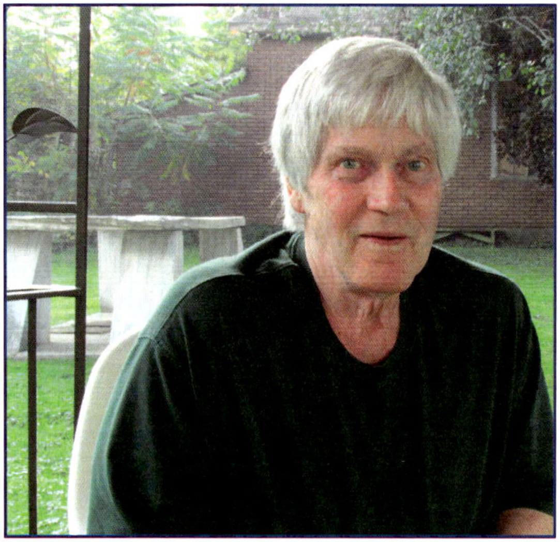

Few stories illustrate Rev. Richard Marceau's belief in the power of serendipity, hard work and love to together facilitate healing better than that of Brian Cavanaugh. After Cavanaugh's car accident 28 years ago, he, like so many other persons profiled in this book, was at first considered dead, then, after he awoke from a five-day coma, not expected to function again on his own. Today, he is a life-skills aide at Lenny Burke's Farm, a dedicated husband, and an avid reader and student of Buddhism, which he says helps him to stay calm when frustration, the result of his head injury, could easily turn to anger.

Cavanaugh, who lives in Pittsford, Vermont, had been drinking at home one night in 1986 when one of his dogs took off; he put the other two in the bed of his pick-up truck and went looking for the dog. He says he must have fallen asleep or blacked out because his vehicle crossed Route 7 into the other lane where "a tractor trailer ran me over." While both dogs died, Cavanaugh says he must have slumped over to one side because the engine block went through the cab of his truck, narrowly missing crushing him. His injuries were so severe that at first he was not expected to survive.

In 1986, little was known about how to care for people with traumatic brain injuries. Cavanaugh received therapy for a badly fractured hip and other physical injuries but minimal cognitive rehabilitation after he awoke from his coma. After a long hospitalization in Rutland, little of which he remembers, he was transferred to the Veterans Administration hospital in White River Junction, where he had extensive physical therapy for another six months.

All the while, his wife, Kay Cavanaugh, a person who, although legally blind, has worked as a medical transcriptionist at the Rutland Hospital for 38 years, "stuck with me. When I came home from White River Junction, they never said anything about what problems I might have. Nothing. I was totally unaware of my problems. I was in a fog. I didn't have a car. Kay doesn't drive. My brother bought me a bicycle, which I rode for quite a while. And then an old friend gave me an old car and the job I used to have in Middlebury at Agri-Mark called me back. This was a job I'd done for six or seven years. I couldn't do it. Then the anger went sky-high because I couldn't do the things I used to do. I'd been totally unprepared for that."

Cavanaugh had grown up with a father who, although he had no education, had never missed a day of work in his life. He felt useless not being able to work.

Meanwhile, somehow, Emmie Burke had heard of Cavanaugh and put him on her mailing list for support group meetings that she, Dr. Ron Savage and

Reverend Marceau were organizing for people who had sustained brain injuries. "I didn't pay attention to it at first but then there was a conference at the Cortina Inn and I went to that," he recalls. There, he met Emmie and Rev and Lenny and things began to come together; he began to see that his anger and frustration were the result of his brain injury. He started attending meetings regularly and then a conference organized by the Head Injury/Stroke Independence Project with Dr. Thomas McAllister, a leading TBI authority from Dartmouth-Hitchcock, as the keynote speaker.

"He was speaking right to me," Cavanaugh recalls. "I was flabbergasted. I told Rev I have got to talk to this man. Rev got me an appointment with him, just like that." When Cavanaugh met with McAllister, he says the doctor couldn't believe he'd functioned so well without medical support and medication. The doctor discovered that Cavanaugh's adrenaline level was off the charts. Once he was treated for that, "I've been fine since. It's not that I don't get mad, like anyone else; I just don't lose control."

Cavanaugh eventually got a job through the state Department of Vocational Rehabilitation with Vermont Tubbs, where his boss helped devise work assignments that he could do because they involved repetitive acts. He says his boss, Ira Colby, told him that, despite his brain injury, "It's better for me to hire you because I know you'll work harder than the next guy. You really want a job."

Cavanaugh had the job for 10 years before Colby left Tubbs and the new boss let him go when he couldn't perform more complicated tasks. Meanwhile, Cavanaugh had been attending support meetings and services at the Church of the Wildwood, where Rev was the minister. One day, Rev asked how work was going. Cavanaugh explained what had happened.

"A week later, he called me at home. 'Brian, would you like to try working at the farm?' he said. I hesitated. 'Just try,' he said. That was 13 years ago and I've been here ever since. I believe by doing the repetitious work for so long that it stimulated my brain to where I could multitask. I'm much better now. It took a long time, but my memory came back," he says. "All along, I could've collected disability but I wanted to work."

Cavanaugh's life is also a good example as to how people's expectations of you can affect your capabilities. While Rev believed Cavanaugh could hold a job that required multiple skills, he had a less fortunate experience while at the VA hospital, one that in turn was countered by someone he met while working at Tubbs. Here's the story:

While Cavanaugh was at the VA hospital, he took a book out of the library and had it beside him in his wheelchair. A nurse asked why he had taken it and he naturally replied that he was going to read it. He recalls her answer to this day: "Brian, you can't read any more."

"So I figured I couldn't, she should know, right? That's a terrible thing to say that I didn't try, but I thought she knew my limitations," he says.

Fortunately, while he was at Tubbs, the company enrolled in a state program in which reading specialists worked with employees who had reading disabilities for an hour or so each week. Cavanaugh recalls his reading instructor telling him, "'Brian, the only thing you need to do to read is read, read, read. Read newspapers to start. A little at a time.' That's exactly what I did. Then she had me write stream of consciousness. It took quite a while but now I can write and read fine."

Among the books that the state reading specialist brought in were ones on Buddhism and they caught Cavanaugh's attention. "That's what I've been reading ever since," he says, adding that the philosophy of

Buddhism and practice of meditation help him control his frustration with what he cannot do and help him to stay focused.

Now 68 years old, Cavanaugh says, "I ask myself, why am I not like the ones that are more badly injured. I have to give credit to my wife. A lot of men with TBIs lose their wives. My wife has always been there 100 percent of the way. One hand washes the other. I have the eyes and take her anywhere she has to go and she supports me in the ways that I need help. We are a team and it's made all the difference for me, having her support all along the way."

And then he speaks of another woman whose dedication has made a difference in his life.

"From the moment I came to the farm, I saw that Lenny is very compassionate, the way his mother is. He has empathy and insight beyond what a lot of people with TBI have. What she did with him and this farm, it's almost unfathomable what one person can do. It's because she operated as a woman, a woman and a mother. It's that combination of compassion and thinking outside the box, bringing commonsense to a problem and never giving up. It takes a very special person to do that and she's done it so well."

And then he adds, "And yet they have men as presidents."

Moderate & severe head injury (respectively) is associated with a 2.3 and 4.5 times increased risk of Alzheimer's disease.

Jean McDuff

Researchers tell us that a person who has sustained a traumatic brain injury is more likely to sustain another than someone who has not. But that, according to Jean McDuff, is not something that should keep you from having a good life. Indeed, McDuff, a man who speaks two languages well – English and Quebecois French – is living proof of a rewarding life despite two quite separate injuries to his head.

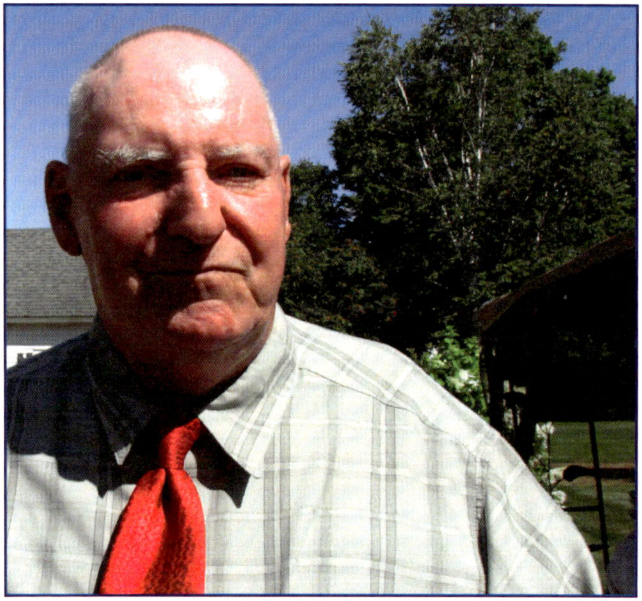

Born to parents who lived in Quebec, where he spoke French primarily, McDuff and his family moved to Island Pond, Vermont, when he was five years old. Two years later, he was diagnosed with a brain tumor. After surgery and a lengthy hospitalization, he was left with paralysis on his left side. He attended the Vermont Achievement Center

for a year, then returned to regular school in his hometown, but went to VAC in the summer. Each year, his teachers noted improvement. As his one-on-one aide, Gary Miller-Wade puts it, "Don't tell Jean he can't do something."

Indeed. As an adult, McDuff wanted to work in a cheese-making plant in Huntington but to do so one needed the use of one's arms and legs, both of them … or so people thought. He kept applying for a job at the local cheese factory and eventually got an interview and a trial job as a shredder. One of his bosses gave him two weeks to last then took a job in Boston. Fifteen years later, the man came back and McDuff was the head cheesemaker. And if you ever want to know anything about the quality of cheese or how to make it, he's the man to ask.

In January 2000, after 20 years, McDuff retired from the cheese company Jolina Foods and moved to the Bardwell House in Rutland, which has assisted living apartments. Due to the paralysis and the special shoes and braces he wears – they weigh a lot! – he felt more secure living there. However, one day three years ago, he was coming out of the movies at the nearby theater when a woman backing up didn't see him and hit him. He fell and hit his head on the concrete. Now, a second injury and a coma. He was in the Rutland Hospital for nine weeks.

"I was sleeping a lot, aware and not aware. I had some memory loss and my body was still weak," he recalls. When it was time to be released, his family members and the nurses urged him not to go home to his apartment where he would be alone. And, thus, McDuff, the old cheesemaker, the Quebecois, found himself living at Lenny Burke's Farm.

"He fought hard all through his recovery," Miller-Wade says. "He would go up and down the stairs at the farm over and over, building up his strength."

Adds McDuff, "I had to write everything on a paper every day, keep a journal. And eventually my memory got better – although it's not perfect."

Today, at 62, he's back in his neat apartment, decorated with dozens of mobiles and the photographs of relatives. McDuff volunteers as a courier at the Rutland Hospital, which means he gets up at 4 a.m., catches the bus and is at the hospital by 6 a.m. There he delivers material from one department to the other. And, so he won't lose the ability to write the Quebecois his grandmother taught him as a child, he still writes his 87-year-old mother each week.

And he's teaching Miller-Wade to speak French.

Males are about twice as likely as females to experience a TBI.

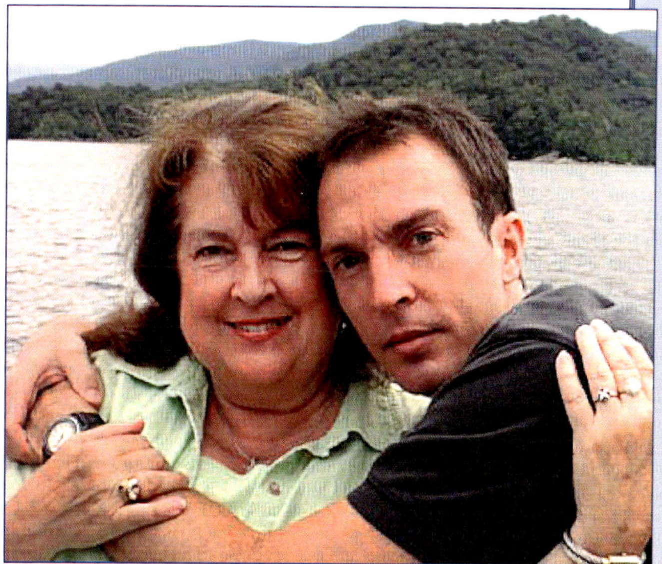

Michael Burke with his mother Emmie on a recent visit home.

seemed to be reaching out to him, Lenny faced a long recovery. He would have to learn basic skills from feeding and grooming himself to more complex actions such as making decisions. He would have to undergo countless hours of therapy to regain strength, especially on his left side, which was primarily affected by the head injury. Also, the boy with perfect vision, a gift to any athlete and one he had taken for granted, now had one normal eye and the other, the left, misaligned, the resulting depth perception adding to his coordination problems. Most daunting would be coming to terms with the fact that he was not the same physically or mentally as the boy who had gone up for that layup shot.

Fortunately, Kathy and her friends were young enough that they knew how to have fun even under these difficult conditions and they enjoyed turning Lenny's therapy into play. Lenny loved singing. Kathy had a microphone and speakers and would give the mike to Lenny, suggest a song, and then shout, "Hit it, Lenny." As a pianist, Emmie certainly understood the power of music and song, but when she heard her son recall words to songs with so much ease, she began to see music as a therapeutic tool. Being the inveterate student, she did her research and discovered that the ability to sing resides in a different part of the brain from language. Most of us have stored the words to songs we haven't sung in years. This was something she and Kathy discovered quite by chance as Lenny belted out the words to both childhood and popular songs. "Kathy became like the little therapist," says Emmie. "Her ideas were like play but it was play that had big results."

One continuing problem, however, was that the shunt in Lenny's head had become infected and needed to be removed. But this, too, could present life-threatening problems. Humans are born with a shunt in their brain, which allows the natural flow of fluid through the head, but Upton had no way of knowing whether Lenny's natural drainage system would take over. It needed to work immediately after the artificial one was removed or he could die. Eventually, he had no choice. The surgery was done on June 1 with Upton strongly requesting that Emmie not let anyone outside the family know about it. He didn't want to "upset the girls." Lenny still had quite a following among the teenage girls and the nursing staff at the hospital and each procedure caused an avalanche of phone calls to the hospital. There were no problems.

About this time, Lenny started regular physical therapy treatments at the Vermont Achievement Center in Rutland, a service and training facility that helps individuals with all manner of disabilities. All that summer, he worked out on a universal gym at Mount St. Joseph under the supervision of his basketball coach Jim Kelley. Emmie worked out with him, too. Today, she laughs as she recalls the shape she was in, charging up and down the bleachers, running in circles and shooting hoops with her son, practicing the monster drills that Lenny used to do with his basketball team.

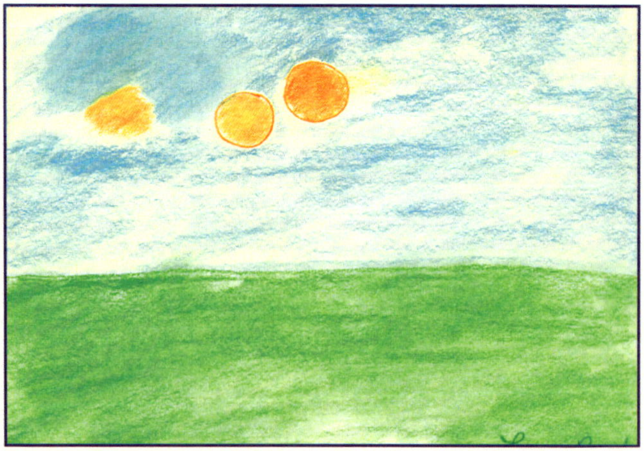

Lenny's painting, "Three Suns."

It wasn't all physical exercise. At home, Emmie was working on intellectual exercise of the most basic kind, tedious work to retrain Lenny's brain. Again, going on instinct, she started at the beginning, giving him crayons and colored pencils and paper, playing word and matching games and designing a strict schedule to help keep him learning. Lenny's drawings often elicited an emotional response from those who saw them. In one there are three suns, which he identified as Jesus, Mother Mary, and Lenny. Today, the drawing is framed and displayed in the family living room. When Lenny pointed it out recently, he said his was the smallest and misshapen sun because he was "the imperfect one." In another rather prophetic picture, Lenny drew a farm scene, complete with rolling hills and a barn, saying to his mom, "Maybe we'll live in a place like that some day and maybe you can help other people like me."

Throughout Lenny's early recovery, Emmie and her friends, John and Marion Austin, had developed a deep curiosity about the treatment of head injuries and strokes and took every opportunity to communicate with people nationwide who specialized in the study of the brain. Thus, in July, 1979, Emmie and Len, accompanied by the Austins, decided to attend a conference on brain injury and stroke organized for professionals in the field and held in neighboring New Hampshire.

Among the presenters were therapists from Rancho Los Amigos, an organization located in Downey, California, that specializes in the treatment and rehabilitation of people with severe brain trauma and other disabling conditions.

Danese Malkmus, the language and speech pathologist at Rancho, and others from the organization had never had parents attend a professional conference before and later told Emmie they had spent the night before their presentation adjusting their talk. They were afraid that their blunt and honest descriptions of the challenges faced by people with severe brain trauma might upset them. At the same time, the Rancho Los Amigos therapists were impressed by Emmie's interest and lay understanding of the subject. Toward the end of the conference, Malkmus gave Emmie her business card and suggested that if problems developed working with Lenny at home she consider bringing him to Rancho Los Amigos. This was an unusual offer because the center usually worked with individuals as soon after their injuries as possible, when the most productive rehabilitation could occur, rather than months later.

"It was apparent that I was doing what they (the therapists) were doing, providing Lenny with a daily structure. It just made sense to me that if he had known these things when he was a child, he could learn them again, that the skills were still in his brain but he was having difficulty retrieving them. I also know that the way we learn how to do things like tie our shoes or ride a bike comes from trial and error and repetition. So, I applied that understanding to re-teaching Lenny. I would take Polaroid photos every day as we got dressed or did household chores and we would go over the photos the next day, discussing everything that Lenny had done the previous day. We'd look at the clothes he was wearing compared to what he had worn the day before," Emmie recalls. "We'd talk about what he had eaten the day before, then make a plan for that day's meals. It was recovery, recovery, recovery; repetition, repetition, repetition."

The routine began with dressing and then breakfast at the same time every day, Captain Crunch, of course, with Lenny setting the table. "I've been setting the table since I was six years old," Lenny says, smiling his beatific grin, "and believe it or not, I liked doing it. I still do. That's because I like to eat."

David Coffman and Liz Doe: A Love Story

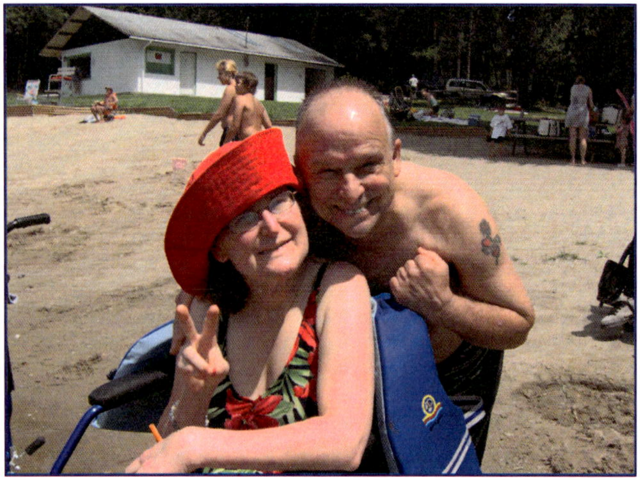

Elizabeth Doe and David Coffman at Elfin Lake in Wallingford. The Rev. Richard Marceau celebrated their "life commitment" service several years before her death in 2012.

David Coffman and Liz Doe's romance seems an unlikely story, considering that both sustained serious brain injuries, Coffman when he was only 12 years old and living in South Carolina, and Doe when she was 20 and living in Arizona. The two travelled separate and somewhat convoluted routes before ending up at Lenny Burke's Farm and finding one another.

Coffman was simply coming out of school when he was hit by a car as he crossed the street. Born in Bermuda to a military father and his wife, Coffman had lived in Spain and Germany before then. The collision caused severe damage to his brainstem and a badly mangled leg. Coffman turned 13 while in a coma, which lasted nearly three months. As a child he'd had severe asthma, which was exacerbated by the long hospitalization.

His sister, Elizabeth Fessler, is 10 years older than him and was already married at the time. She understands how tragic the accident was as Coffman was a very bright child who still remembers words in the five or six languages he learned during his travels as a child. He's still capable of reading and understanding, she says, but his growth and maturity, as with many people who sustain brain injuries, was seriously affected by the injury to his brain.

"When he got out of the hospital, he was incapable of doing anything for himself. Our mother spent a year getting him to walk, talk, dress himself. She stayed with him all the time, like having a baby. Our parents decided to relocate to Franklin, Vermont, and tried to put him in Missisquoi Union High School, but that didn't work. That's where he discovered his losses," she says.

As an adult, Coffman spent a few years at the Crotched Mountain Rehabilitation Center before a caregiver recommended that he move to Lenny Burke's Farm. Says Fessler: "It was almost too good to be true. He loves people, loves to draw, loves to write poems and love songs. It was the perfect fit. When he fell in love with Liz, he would write her songs and record them so she could listen to them, especially later when she was sick. He's stabilized now; he's maturing. His injury affected his short-term memory but his long-term memory has remained very good. While at the farm, his brain has been able to almost re-circuit itself and he has expanded his memory of the past and improved his short-term memory.

"David loves church. He loved Rev and took Rev's death quite hard. Rev did the commitment of love ceremony for David and Liz, which was so important to both of them. For people who have lost so much, that celebration was reaffirming. Her death was hard, too, but he believes she's in heaven and at peace and that he'll join her there some day."

Liz's real name is Elizabeth Doe. Her mother, Judy Gray, was originally from the Brattleboro, Vermont, area but now lives in West Palm Beach, Florida. Gray was 20 when she gave her daughter up for adoption to a family whose last name was Doe.

Doe was raised in Arizona where her adoptive father was an airplane pilot. In 1989, when Doe was just 20, she was hit by a car while riding her bicycle and thrown into a concrete draining ditch. Besides devastating damage to her left leg and foot, she was in a coma for several months and also sustained damage to her pancreas, which led to her having diabetes. As her mother puts it, she was "pretty well destroyed."

After her rehabilitation, she lived with her adoptive parents until her adoptive mother passed away in 1997 and the adoptive father, who was quite elderly, remarried. Enter Gray's other daughter, who'd also been adopted; Gray had found her in 1989 just before Doe's accident. Together the two discovered that Doe was in a nursing home in Arizona. Gray was able to gain guardianship of her, "trucked her back to Vermont and didn't have a clue what to do after that. All I knew was that she didn't belong in a nursing home. I had her home for about six weeks before I, too, hard as it was, placed her in a nursing home. Then, through the state of Vermont I found out about Lenny Burke's Farm. Hallelujah."

"The strides she made after going there were amazing. I'm so thankful that Elizabeth had that the last 14 years of her life," says Gray, who is especially fond of Kathy Chandler. "She made my daughter's life and her final months the best, as close to a full life as possible. And I am so glad she had a relationship, someone to love in David, before she died. I lament the years I didn't have her, but I'm happy I was able to help her when she needed help the most."

According to Chandler, Doe had many struggles with illnesses and was frequently hospitalized after moving to Vermont. Chandler or another staff member would stay with her when she had to be hospitalized. Besides the diabetes and other problems, she was diagnosed with throat cancer in 2012.

"She wanted to die at home and so we brought her home and she was with us for the final days. Hospice was wonderful. It was very meaningful to all the clients to have her here; she'd been with us for so long. I cleared my schedule and spent my time with Liz, letting her eat food she couldn't normally eat. We prettied her up, put jewelry on her, put flowers in her room. David visited often. On her last day, the sun was shining. Kevin (Burke) came over and they had a lovely visit. It was a perfect day.

"At one point, I asked her, 'Is there anything you want? You know what's going on?' And she said, 'I have cancer and I'm dying. I'm scared. I'm worried about David.'

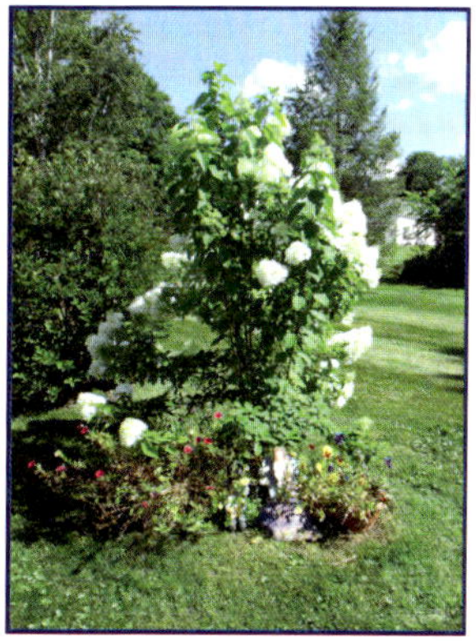

"I said, 'You are? You know what I am,' and she said, 'Yeah, you're my sis, my best friend.' And I said, 'Yes, but I'm also the boss of this house and I'm going to make sure that David gets taken care of. I don't want you to worry about that. If you have pain you tell me. The world is your oyster today. Don't be afraid. We'll take care of everything. It's not going to be long.' She hugged me. We cried. And the next morning at 7 a.m. she died."

Liz's ashes are buried at Lenny Burke's Farm, where David Coffman visits the tree planted above them. He sits and sings the songs he wrote for her.

"She's my angel and I'll be with her someday," he said last summer as the hydrangea tree planted in her memory was in full bloom.

Indeed, knowing that Lenny enjoyed eating as much after his injury as before, Emmie used Lenny's love of food as a learning tool. After the injury to his brain, Lenny's left arm was contracted so that it was bent a little backward at the elbow and almost frozen at an awkward angle. For months he had worn a cast to help straighten it out; the cast had worked only partway and he avoided using this arm. Fortunately, it was Lenny's left arm, not the right. Emmie was convinced that she could improve its flexibility. She had kept the cast and came up with the idea of putting it on Lenny's good arm – the right one – so that when he did routine tasks like setting the table, he had to use the left arm, the one he didn't like using. She would let him eat with his right arm but when it came to dessert, especially ice cream, she would put the cast on the right arm so that he had to use the left. Over time, the arm and the coordination improved.

"Because he loved food so much, we'd take photos of what he'd eaten, over and over training or retraining his brain to remember what he'd done the day before and the day before that, then repeating much of it for that day or saying, 'No, we had that on Tuesday, remember? What haven't we had for lunch in a while?' We did dots to dots, played word searches. Because his eye was so deviated, he had tunnel vision and would only see what was right in front of him. He had to physically move his head to see something to the side. I worked for hours on his peripheral vision, on getting him to see more broadly. Lenny loves sweets so I put M & Ms all around his desk. He would have to scan the desk to find the candy. I would hide his favorite foods so he'd have to go look for them. I hid money all around his room and told him to go look for it. Of course, now there's nothing he can't find."

Eventually, over the course of many weeks, Lenny's eye muscles got stronger and stronger and the deviation decreased. One of Upton's major surprises was the day he observed that Lenny's eye had gone back to its natural position, something he did not think would happen.

For each of these daily tasks, there was often a test. Emmie would say, "'Lenny, close your eyes and tell me what you are wearing.' Sometimes he'd have to look to tell me but that was okay because in repeating it, he was exercising his memory." One day when Lenny was at Upton's office for a physical, Upton told Lenny to close his eyes before checking his reflexes. Lenny quite automatically answered, "Blue jeans, red and green shirt, white sneakers."

All this was well and good but Emmie had begun to realize that this tough routine was in danger of damaging the mother/son relationship she had with Lenny. Everything was a learning experience – and this was good – but when could the two of them just relax and let the lessons go for a little while? She worried about Kathy, too. Was she getting the attention she needed? Michael and Kevin were older now and involved in their own school activities. Emmie knew she had taken Lenny quite far but she worried that her son needed more professional help to move forward and she didn't want to miss her daughter's pre-teen and early teen years, such an important time between mothers and daughters.

And so Emmie remembered Rancho Los Amigos. Recalling that the center had never had a client as far removed time-wise from his or her injury as Lenny, she asked the Vermont Achievement Center to make tapes of Lenny to show where he was at physically. The therapists at Rancho viewed the tapes and told Emmie that, despite the passage of time, they would accept him as a client. This meant leaving home for several months, a departure that would be particularly hard on Michael who had become quite close to Lenny. The two were very compatible, sharing a quick wit and dry sense of humor. They'd long shared a room and loved to pull practical jokes on their parents, many of them ironically having a dark side, such as pretending to be injured or that they were fighting. Michael recalls the time he and Lenny pretended to have a huge argument complete with fisticuffs. Len and Emmie were in the next room and all they could hear was the sound of fists on skin. As their parents rushed in, Michael took a huge swing at Lenny, who clapped his hands together mimicking the sound of a fist hitting head and then fell to the ground. "My dad almost hit me, thinking I had hurt Lenny," recalls Michael, smiling with the memory of all the pranks he and Lenny had succeeded in pulling off.

One of the things that still impresses Michael about Lenny is how Lenny included both his brothers in so many of his activities and shared his friends with them. "He let me be friends with his friends," says Michael. Of course, back then Michael didn't realize how unusual it was for a high school boy to include a brother who was still in grammar school in his activities.

Michael had not been at the game where Lenny was injured, having decided to hang out with a friend. He made up for that in the weeks and months after Lenny's injury, sitting with him during MSJ's basketball game against its rival Rutland, holding Lenny's hand throughout the game. Like Kathy, he enjoyed taking part in Lenny's rehabilitation. One of the things that amazed him was Lenny's recall for names, dates and events. He'd drill Lenny with questions, curious about what was retained and what was not and often surprised that when it came to people's names or the phone numbers of girls they knew, Lenny's memory was sometimes better than his own.

That said, the pranks didn't end with Lenny's injury. When Lenny had just learned how to walk, Michael was convinced he could still ride a bike, again based on deep memory. He spent an hour or two getting Lenny comfortable on the bike and then called his mother, hoping to surprise her. The minute she came out of the house, Lenny rode down the driveway and whipped into traffic. "We had it planned that way. Mom went from joy to terror. That's how we treated her as kids," says Michael, realizing as an adult how his mother must have felt.

At the time of the planned trip to Rancho Los Amigos, Kevin was a junior in high school and Michael was in junior high. The two promised to hold down the fort while their mom was gone and to stay out of trouble (a promise they readily admit today that they didn't keep. As Michael puts it, "We took advantage of our parents' distraction.")

Emmie had decided that Kathy, then 11, would accompany her and Lenny to California. Like Emmie, Kathy had a strong sense of responsibility; Emmie knew it would be Kathy who would be doing much of the housework if she were the only female at home. And, besides, taking Kathy with her would allow the two to have special time while Lenny was sleeping or in therapy sessions. Kathy brought her schoolwork with her and Marion and John Austin's daughter Gail, who had often stayed at the Burkes' to help Emmie around the house, offered to travel with them and keep Kathy company when Emmie was at the center with Lenny.

Of course, Len would be home with the boys, but Lenny's injury and Emmie's growing independence had caused a change in him, too. He just couldn't seem to shake his sorrow over Lenny's diminished

Jason O'Connor: Nature Boy

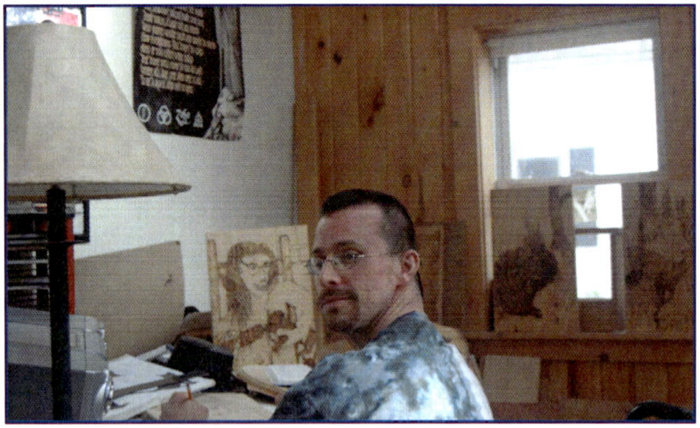

Jason O'Connor in his room surrounded by some of his artwork.

One gets the sense that Jason O'Connor has always been a handful, an energetic kid who loved to swim, play in the woods and, occasionally, try his parents' patience. At 38, he has the same impish grin he had when he was a boy, a look that telegraphs energy and independence. He had just celebrated his 12th birthday and was at his grandmother's to celebrate his mom's birthday on June 17, 1988 when, without looking, he ran into the road and was hit by a car.

His coma lasted all summer. Paula O'Connor reminds one of Emmie Burke. She too began educating herself about head injuries and worked with doctors and therapists at Rhode Island Hospital immediately after her son's injury to try to keep his muscles from atrophying.

The damage to O'Connor's brain and body was so extensive that he was transferred to the Braintree Rehabilitation Center in Braintree, Mass, where he underwent extensive speech, occupational and physical therapy for months before being sent home.

At that point, O'Connor couldn't stand on his own; indeed, his balance was so bad he had to be supported even when in a sitting position. He was right-handed and his right side was paralyzed with his arm, somewhat like Lenny's, almost frozen in an upright position.

Through his school district in North Kingston, R.I., O'Connor was enrolled in the Sargent Rehabilitation Center, where he took classes. After school, his mother took him for three more hours of rehabilitation and education. O'Connor's family lives on a property with an Olympic style swimming pool; swimming was one of the things O'Connor could do after the accident. His mother also enrolled him in sailing and horseback riding programs, which, over time, enabled him to regain balance. She explains that a horse's gait, hip to hip, is similar to the human's and often used in therapy for people with head injuries.

It was a private therapist, Janice Hulme, who got him up on his feet. Paula O'Connor remembers Hulme's first meeting and evaluation with her son after which she told her husband, "'Guess what? God is a woman.' That's how much she affected me."

Over time, O'Connor progressed from a wheelchair to a walker. He can walk a bit on his own now and is quite adept at getting downstairs on his butt or otherwise maneuvering his body from place to place.

Taking her son to his various therapies was a fulltime job for Paula O'Connor whose husband Jack ran his own business. She concedes a younger daughter, Erin, suffered from the amount of time given to Jason but he eventually graduated from high school at age 21, receiving a standing ovation as he walked on his own to get his diploma.

Caring for him, however, had taken a toll and, with the loss of the Sargent program, the family began looking for a residential setting for O'Connor. Paula

O'Connor had been active for years in the Brain Injury Association of Rhode Island, a branch of the national organization; she stepped down after serving in a number of positions including president two years ago.

Through the organization, she met the parents of Meredith Coffey and Daniel Fanning, two Rhode Island residents already living at Lenny Burke's Farm. When she dropped her son off for his evaluation, he immediately told Emmie and Rev not to get too attached; his parents would be back to get him in two weeks.

Before the two weeks were up, though, he'd worked with some of the farm animals and made the acquaintance of two men connected with the farm – Butch Towsley and Gary Jaquith. Towsley worked with clients at the farm doing this and that. He and O'Connor got talking about fishing and hunting and, before long, Towsley invited him to his camp in nearby Tinmouth. Fishing and swimming? Well, that wasn't half bad.

Jaquith shared O'Connor's love of animals and would talk with him for hours.

When O'Connor's two-week trial period was over, he announced no way was he going back to Rhode Island.

Even before arriving at the farm, O'Connor had been splitting wood for spending money. As a boy, he'd shown artistic ability and this led his mother to buy a wood-burning kit, thinking he might be able to use it with his left hand. Indeed, he could.

He was a handful for his mother in the last year he was home, frustrated with what he couldn't do. He had a part-time job at Chicago Pizza folding boxes, emptying the trash and cleaning up. But he wanted the kind of physical activity that, without help, the family could not provide.

He was a handful, too, when he arrived at Lenny Burke's Farm. They used a lift to bring him upstairs to his room but he quickly learned to scoot down on his butt when he was supposed to be sleeping. Emmie, whose room was below his, would keep one eye and one ear open all night to keep track of him.

But watching him try and try to do some task like make pizza on his own impressed her so much; she thought, "My god, he tries so hard. I've got to find people who will help him." Towsley, of course, was the perfect fit. O'Connor wanted to learn how to hunt and to fish. Towsley taught him how to use a crossbow. He took him fishing on Tinmouth Pond. All the while, O'Connor worked out on weights, building his upper body muscles.

These days, he uses that upper body strength to split wood he often gets from Towsley, primarily using his left hand and arm with the axe. He piles the wood on his wheelchair seat and using the arm rests for ballast, uses the wheelchair to move the wood to where he plans to stack it for sale. He uses the money he makes to go to concerts with another aide, Jim Fleshman. At group meetings when clients gather to talk and sing together, O'Connor always chooses something by Led Zeppelin.

Emmie is particularly fond of him, saying, "I got to know him really well. He'd be watching TV at night and he would holler to me, 'Emmie, The Golden Girls are on. Emmie, there's something about women on the TV you might like.' He loves to talk, loves history, especially stuff about wars. He's so bright and personable, we got very close."

A few years ago, hearing O'Connor wax poetic about wanting to live by himself in a log cabin, Emmie had the bottom of the barn located at Emma's Place made into an apartment for O'Connor, complete with pine wood walls. He proudly shows off his wood-burning tools, barbells, the toys he purchases for the latest of his precious cats, like all the others over the years named Cosmo, and dozens of pieces of art that he's made. The latest is of a cat that resembles Cosmo.

And, after all these years, while O'Connor loves going home for Thanksgiving, Christmas, Easter and a summer vacation, he says, "I love it here. It's home. I'm so glad I stayed."

> "The greatest discovery of any generation is that a human can alter his life by altering his attitude."
>
> *—William James*

"If You Change Your Mind, You Change Your Life."

(Editor's note: The Rev. Richard Marceau was an integral part of Lenny Burke's Farm from its inception until his death in 2010. This excerpt from a keynote talk he gave at an annual TBI conference is an example of what he brought to the community of people who have experienced a traumatic brain injury, their families and friends, and people who treat them.)

There's a certain, very special energy here at the conferences, when we come together each year. Nineteen years. We have come a long, long ways.

Serendipity is just a wonderful thing, just one of the things that are going to touch you one way or the other, today. Before you leave.

Em, I've kind of calculated that over the past twenty years I've spent well in excess of a thousand hours in meetings and groups and circles of people who have experienced a traumatic brain injury. And in those hundreds and hundreds and hundreds of hours, we've cried together, we have laughed together, we have mourned deep deep losses together … but most of all we celebrate.

We celebrate the tiniest little steps forward as victories. As moving forward to the healing of the whole person. No step forward is too small to be acknowledged, and to be celebrated.

I want to share with you some of the things that I have seen, some of the miracles that I have seen in recovery, things I have learned about recovery and traumatic brain injury. And even though I share them with you, these things that are specific to TBI, I think they have to do with just being a human being. Because what's true about being a human being, TBI or not, is it's not what happens to us that makes a difference, it's how we choose to respond to it.

Think that's true?

It's not what happened to me, it's how I choose to respond to it.

Two people can experience the exact same thing and have totally different responses. One gets bitter and one gets better. Have you seen that?

I have a lot of heroes, and people that I admire. One of them was Max Cleland. I'm sure you know his story. He was a young captain in the Air Force in the Vietnam War. He rotated out, went far away from home and, while he was out in the jungle one day with his men, flying in and out of the jungle, a situation arose, and wanting to protect his men, he jumped on a grenade and it wasn't to be that he was okay … and it went off.

He lost both legs and one arm. And when he was in rehab, he went through a dark, dark time. He entered a deep, dark depression. What kind of a life could a man live with no legs? With one arm?

He discovered that life as he knew it was over.

But out of that darkness, one night he had an epiphany.

Do you know what an epiphany is? Have you ever had that?

When all of a sudden a light goes off within you? An ah-ha! moment in time, an epiphany? You suddenly know something new.

Wait a minute here! I'm not my arms, or my legs, or even my body … I am so much more than that! I am still alive. I am the ME that lives in my mind and that ME is still alive, and I can become a new ME.

And to make a long story short, a few years later, he stood in front of a joint session of the United States Congress and was introduced as the director of services in the Veterans Administration, and received a standing ovation. He went on from there to become the senator, the United States senator, from the state of Georgia.

He changed his mind, he changed the way he responded, and everything changed.

It's not what happens to you and me; it's how we choose to respond to it.

Makes all the difference in the world.

I want to tell you about someone else today, a person named Brian. He's given me permission to tell his story. Brian had a traumatic injury about 20 years ago … a head-on collision when a tractor-trailer hit him in a small pickup … and over those 20 years he went through darkness. He went through struggle and depression.

He went through anger and rage. He went through struggling with relationships. The circumstances led to much anger and rage about failures in work and vocation.

And Brian had an epiphany. Believe it or not he had one right here at one of these conferences.

You never know what is going to happen.

He met and found Dr. McAllister and he started attending some of our groups after a while. Brian changed his mind. He started changing the way he responded to what happened to him.

I love to hear Brian in group, when he shares with the newly injured.

He says, "I don't call what happened to me in that accident a tragedy, I call it a turning point – a turning point – because I have become a new me and you know what? I love the new me and, as hard as it has been, I saw that I can't imagine becoming what I've become in any other way, without the traumatic brain injury. It may have been one of the best things that ever happened to me in my life."

What do you think of that?

Brian changed his mind, he changed his response, he changed his life.

It's not what happens.

It's how we respond.

Change your mind … change your life.

I'm proud to say that he's now an LSA, life skills aide and caregiver on our staff who was named the Caregiver of the Year right here a few years ago.

It's not what happens, it's how we respond.

William James, who was a professor at Harvard, in the early twentieth century, and who was thought of as the father of modern psychology, said in one of his little books, "The greatest discovery of any generation is that a human can alter his life by altering his attitude."

I pray and I hope that you are able to see that. That you can see the link …I love the title of this year's conference, Meaningful Links. There is a meaningful link between what's happening in your mind and what is happening in your life.

There's a meaningful link, between what's happening in your mind … and in your life. There are a few things we say over and over in our groups. Thoughts are things; thoughts are seeds. What I plant is what grows. If I plant corn and I get corn I'm happy. If I plant corn and I'm looking for watermelon, I'm going to be disappointed. The thoughts I give time and space to in my mind are going to produce outcomes. Where my mind goes, my personal power flows.

I can't control most of the circumstances swirling around me but I can control my responses and my thoughts. There's a meaningful link between the thoughts we give time and space to and what is unfolding in our lives.

One of the stories I tell is of a young Native American brave. He finished his vision quest, and came back to the council to the great chief. And as he sat there he realized he wanted to know more of the meanings of life. He said to the chief, "Could you tell some of the meanings of life?"

"My son, I tell you, for every human being there is a battle that goes on within us. There are two dogs within, two dogs within everybody. There is a white dog that is full of hope and love and honor and bravery and courage. And there is a black dog that is dark and angry and hopeless … and those two dogs are battling all the time within us."

And then there was silence.

Then the young brave said to the great chief, "Who wins the battle?"

And he said, "My son, whichever dog you feed the most."

When I sit in circles with people with traumatic brain injury, week after week, year after year after year, I'm constantly saying that I just want to refuse to call you "survivors." Because surviving isn't enough, surviving is defined as continuing to exist. There's got to be more to it than that. Why would we work to just survive if that's all there is?

We've got to, as hard and painful as it is, be aware of how we can, how I can, in the midst of these circumstances … just as they are, AS THEY ARE … not just survive, but THRIVE and grow and expand … and become that new me, like Brian did.

We have to all realize that life isn't easy, is it? That life isn't fair. It's probably not ever fair, is it?

But there's a wonderful, wonderful zen teaching I brought along to share with you: The obstacles are the path. They are the stepping stones to a new perspective, a new way of looking at life.

Think that's true?

Sometimes those stepping stones are covered with muddy water, and you can't see them. And that's when it's good to ask for help, help to see the way, and then take the first step.

After many years of experience with people with disabilities, what I have discovered is that many times in rehab they ask the wrong questions. They're asking, "What's wrong with you? How can we fix it? And for heaven's sake, what are we going to do with you if we can't fix you?"

Now that's not what we want to ask of our people … The questions we want to ask of our people are: What's RIGHT with you? Where are you strong, even if there's only one strength, and how can we build on it?

The second meaningful link that we have discovered in working in almost twenty years with traumatic brain injury is that we're all recovering from something, aren't we, and that we all want to become whole.

What we know is that it isn't a matter of trying to fix a few deficits that any of us want; it's the healing of the whole person, physically, emotionally, spiritually, relationally, vocationally.

There's a vast difference between being cured and being healed. We can't do it alone. Max wasn't cured, he didn't grow his leg or an arm back … but he was healed. And I think that healing begins with looking in the mirror and coming to accept an absolute truth. "I am a unique, one of a kind person of infinite worth. In the history of the universe there will never be another me.

It's a threefold process to become whole. It involves loving and being loved. A sense that I belong, and that I have a contribution to make

But you can't achieve that alone.

To love and be loved. And I have a contribution to make. And it may not be to earn a living.

You can't achieve that alone. After 25 years, I have come to believe that the only disability that human beings really suffer from is loneliness. Several years ago I saw this on the news, a clip about the Special Olympics. There had been a race with four young men competing, but before the finish one of them fell, fell badly, sprawled right out on the track on his back. The others came back for him. And they dried his tears, and straightened up his shorts and they joined hands … and they walked to the finish line and finished together.

There is a parallel to life here. And there is a parallel to teaching about traumatic brain injury: you cannot do it alone.

Another meaningful link I want to make today is that people are the solution to the problems that confront us. Technology is not the solution, though it certainly can help. We are the solution … We as generous, open-hearted people who want to use our creativity, our caring and compassion and interact with other human beings.

Relationships are all that is. Everything in the universe only exists because it is in relationship with everything else. That's the truth of creation.

We have to stop pretending that we are beings who want to be alone.

Alone is not our natural state.

We only isolate when we've been hurt. We've all been let down by others. Been disappointed. We're going to let that heal. And let that meaningful link of holding hands carry us into the next moment, holding hands as we go together into the future.

To love other people is to let them love you, and to let them love you is to let them know you. Now, that's risky. But the rewards are enormous. That's the truth of creation.

Goals: I hear about them pretty often. "What I want is for things to go back to how it used to be … before I had a traumatic brain injury."

Me too. But we don't have a rewind. This is how it is. This is where I am.

We have to struggle with this painful, painful process and it's hard and it's painful. In the words of Mark Twain, "Denial ain't just a river in Egypt" and boy we struggle with that and it's hard and it's painful and it's hard to have to say, to be able to say that this is the mountain I have to climb and I don't know if I can climb it, that that is the raging river I have to ford. I don't think I can make it .

Maybe together?

It's hard. It's hard. It's hard. It's hard.

The question is … here I am … where do I go from here? Where are the steps I can take? And what do I have to leave behind?

It's okay. You have to grieve the losses. With traumatic brain injury, it's like grieving a death, what might have been … what could have been … and it's okay to be angry, it's okay even to have some despair.

But then we begin to emerge from it. And say, this is where I am. I can't go back. But I can go on.

A meaningful link is not to your past.

A meaningful link takes you to now and to the threshold of your tomorrows.

athletic ability. Yet when therapists said that Lenny would need residential treatment as he got older, Len promised Emmie he would convert their garage into a family room that they could equip with all the machinery Lenny might need so that he could remain at home. And even though he was less than happy that Emmie would be gone for six weeks, he paid for the family to travel to California in mid-March, 1980, buoyed by the hope that the therapists from Rancho Los Amigos might return the old Lenny to him.

As it turned out, the flight west was something of a nightmare. Even though he was excited to be above the clouds and see the world the way Sister Clementine, one of the nuns at MSJ, had described it, Lenny was a mess. The stimulation and activity – not to mention the anticipation – had not set well with him. Lenny had used cream rinse rather than shampoo to wash his hair and that, combined with his halting gait, drew more than unwelcome attention. The flight may have been the first time that Michael, then 13, had observed how strangers reacted to his brother and he was embarrassed for him, a feeling that made him both uncomfortable and protective. "Lenny just looked awful. He was violently sick," Michael recalls. Much as he loved Lenny, Michael was also mortified by the stench of vomit that filled the plane.

Yet, like the other members of his family, as Michael said goodbye to his brother to accompany his father back to Vermont, he was full of hope. "We all thought that he would come back as the old Lenny," he said. "We were sure that they would fix him."

The name of the facility, Rancho Los Amigos, suggests a ranch somewhere in the southwest, open to the weather with horses and rustic cabins. To the contrary, the facility is located near a mall on a busy road, the Imperial Highway, just 17 miles from Los Angeles. The main building is Spanish style but much of the campus looks quite institutional. Lenny, who had only roomed with his brother, now shared a small room with seven strangers. At the time, the center cost $10,000 a month. (Thank heavens for that fundraiser the local community had sponsored.) Emmie, Kathy and Gail lived at a nearby motel run by Indians from South Africa who treated the Burkes like family, cooking delicious, spicy food for them each day.

Recalls Emmie, "They would always say about the food they made for us, 'This is mild,' but it was really hot, delicious but hot. They were the most wonderful people. They were interested in what was happening with Lenny and what was going on at home. They became very involved. The mother dried food on rocks she placed in the sun. She had a jewel in her forehead. This was all very exotic for us. She dressed Gail up in an Indian outfit. They had two beautiful children, Manita and Matish, a boy. They let the kids play with us a lot and loved Kathy so much they wanted to take her to Africa with them when they went to visit. It made being away from home a lot more enjoyable."

Of course, at first the therapists at Rancho Los Amigos didn't want Emmie around during Lenny's rehabilitation sessions. It was quite unusual to have a mother accompany a patient; Lenny was now just shy of 18 and Emmie had already recognized the downside of working so closely with her son. Yet, an idea about sharing what she *and* Lenny had learned about injuries to the brain with others was just beginning to form in her mind, and Emmie, someone who loved learning almost as much as any other pursuit, was hungry to understand this wondrous part of the human body, so essential and yet, even 35 years ago, still quite unexplored.

As it turned out, the therapists soon discovered that Emmie was the only one who could get Lenny to do the most painful or challenging exercises and, thus, they asked her to help with these sessions and allowed her to observe others. It was a tough balancing act and, as she spent more time at Rancho Los Amigos, she began to look for ways to separate Emmie the trainer from Emmie the mother, if that was possible. Yet at the same time, it was evident to her and to the therapists that Emmie had a natural gift in helping people with disabilities. For example, the therapy involved using big balls for balance and confidence: Lenny hated working on these exercise balls and had a hard time getting up on top of them. As encouragement, Emmie would whisper to him how handsome he was and say that when he got home and had all his muscles back, all the girls would swarm all over him. He'd say, "Well, Mom, why don't you get up here and try it."

"We'd have a good laugh about that but I got him to do more and more. They wanted me to tell them what I was saying, but I wouldn't. They probably wouldn't have approved of my methods of motivation. But I knew if you don't have balance, you don't have anything. He gained a lot of trust in every direction doing those exercises, even if the therapists might not have approved of my methods."

Lenny found living in a dormitory with other clients quite difficult as he'd rarely been away from his family. While daytimes were organized with therapy sessions led by the professionals, night times and weekends could be chaotic and scary with just a skeleton crew on duty, many of them distracted by music or the telephone. Even to this day, Lenny will say he trusted his mother but he didn't quite trust the people at Rancho Los Amigos, even the therapists. Fortunately, he was able to spend weekends with the family at the motel – all except one weekend when he wasn't allowed to leave the center as an "incentive" to get him to work harder. That didn't work and wasn't repeated.

The motel was located near a huge mall with a restaurant called Pieloon and Pieloon, of course, specialized in one of Lenny's favorite foods in the world, pie. And not just any pie. "Amazing pies," as Lenny recalls. His favorite: banana cream. Clearly the promise of banana cream pie was a better incentive for Lenny to work harder than threats.

"Those horrible squats to tighten up his gluteus muscles, they were the worst," Emmie says as Lenny groans at even the mention of doing them. "Who knew that the gluteus muscles were such an essential part of movement, such as getting in and out of a car? They're very important. I used to tell him, 'If you are going to court people, you're going to have to squat.' I knew the reward might be better if I put the exercise in that context rather than any other."

It was at Rancho that Emmie fully understood why Lenny could make hoop after hoop when he first came home from the hospital. "They told me he had excellent kinesthetic memory. His physical therapist, Carollee Joyce Winstein, was very capable; after observing Lenny's use of kinesthetic memory and understanding its role in the recovery of people who have had injuries such as his, she went back to school to get her Ph.D in kinesthetic memory. It's simply the memory of the motion of your body. That's why, for a while after Lenny came out of his coma, he was able to shoot hoops effortlessly. He could swish the ball. His left side was still partially paralyzed but he could do it from his memory of the motion.

"The kinesthetic memory helped him a lot as did his therapy in cognitive remediation. I didn't go to these sessions because it would have been too distracting. But I watched the videotapes afterward and saw what they were doing. I felt good about it but it was hard to watch. What he had to do was so tough, really unimaginable, learning to do things

John Shepherd: Out of the Fog

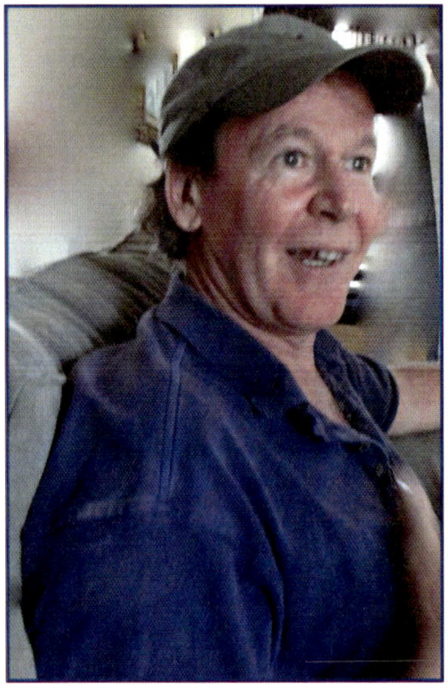

"I was 42 years old for seven years after I had my injury," John Shepherd says by way of explaining the fog he lived in before an employment counselor suggested he attend a conference on brain injury. There, he met Emmie and Kevin Burke and Reverend Marceau and told them his story. "They told me about the farm and said come by and check us out. I came and sat down with Emmie and she hired me to work at the farm," Shepherd recalls.

As the weeks and months progressed, Shepherd's fog retreated and memory returned. He had grown up on a farm so the environment was comfortable. As time progressed and his faculties improved, he began working with clients. Today, he is a life skills aide who works with four men who live on the farm.

In 1999, Shepherd, then 42, was trying to strengthen his back after an injury when he fell off an inversion table, hitting his head on the floor quite hard. He was briefly unconscious but didn't want to go to the hospital. He went to bed to "recover."

That was the beginning of "some really tough times" as, untreated, Shepherd's condition worsened. While his parents wanted him to come home, he was too proud to do so and was homeless for a while, living in a friend's car until another friend offered him a place to stay. Eventually, still struggling with basic needs, he moved to a family home in Arlington, Vermont. That's when he finally got some therapy and learned about brain injury and a conference that might help him get back on track.

Shepherd still lives in Arlington and doesn't drive. He takes the bus to work on Wednesdays, returning home by bus at the end of the week after working some day and some night shifts. "I feel I can understand what the clients are going through because I was in such a fog for a long time. I was so thankful to have been accepted here. It's confirming," he says. "And what I enjoy so much about the farm, this house, and everything about Lenny Burke's Farm, is it's community-based; it's not an institution. I think that's so unique and so healing to have that atmosphere. People here have dignity."

Rancho Los Amigos Levels of Cognitive Functioning

- **Level 1:** No response, person appears to be in deep sleep
- **Level 2:** Generalized response, person reacts inconsistently, not directly in response to stimuli
- **Level 3:** Localized response, reacts inconsistently, directly to stimuli
- **Level 4:** Confused/Agitated, person is extremely confused, agitated
- **Level 5:** Confused-Inappropriate/Non-Agitated, person is confused andresponds inaccurately to commands
- **Level 6:** Confused-Appropriate, Person is confused, responds accurately to commands
- **Level 7:** Automatic-Appropriate, person goes through daily routine with minimal confusion
- **Level 8:** Purposeful-Appropriate, person has functioning memory, responsive to environment, may display depression
- **Level 9:** Purposeful-Appropriate, goes through daily routine aware of need for stand-by assistance, depression may continue
- **Level 10:** Purposeful-Appropriate/Modified Independent, goes through daily routine but may require more time or compensatory strategies, periodic depression may occur.

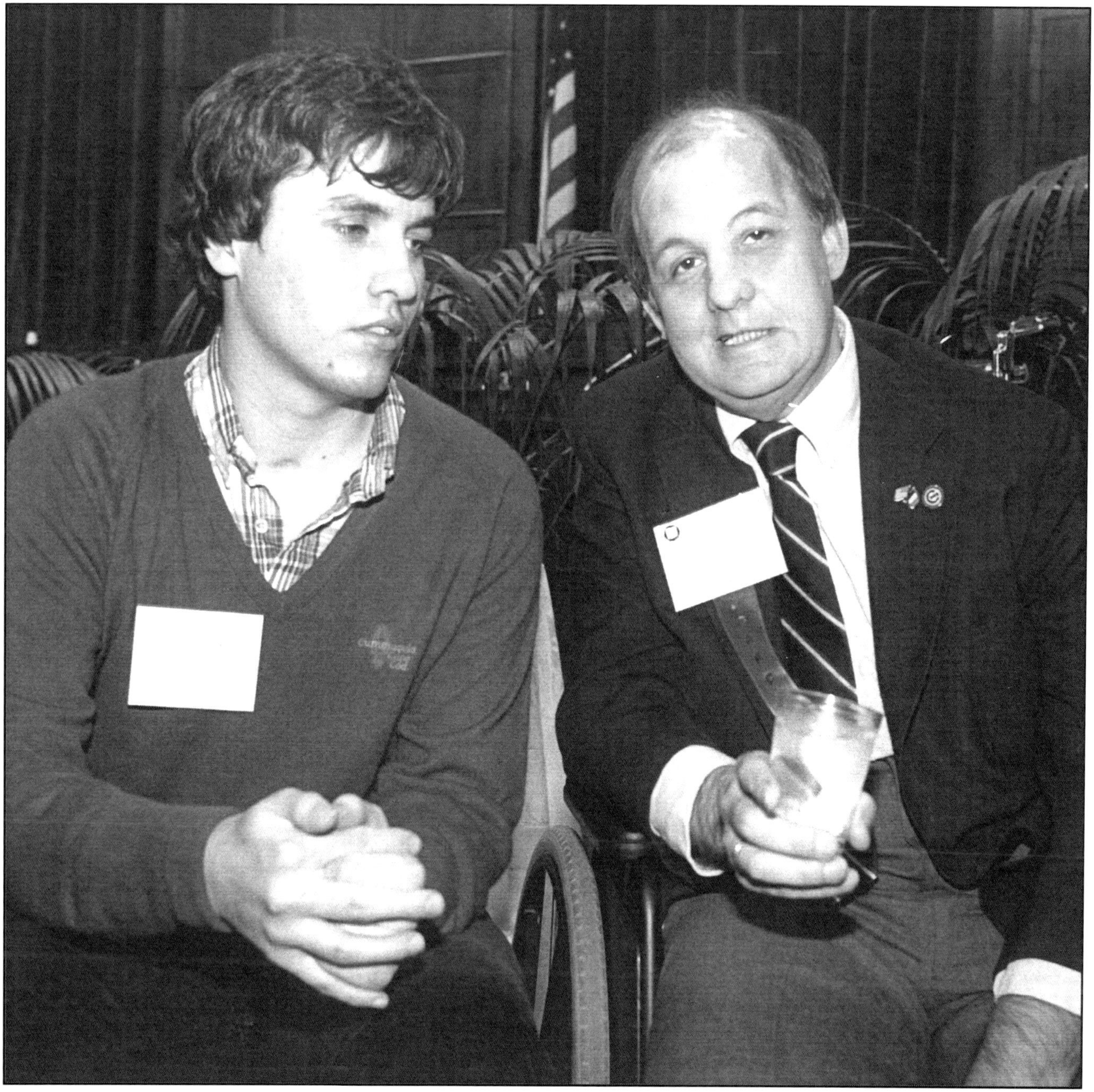

Friends in Rehabilitation: Lenny Burke and James Brady, White House Press Secretary, who sustained a brain injury when he was one of four people shot during John Hinckley's attempted assassination of President Ronald Reagan.

that you used to do without thinking and that you once could do better than anyone else you knew. But most of the time, Lenny had such a great attitude."

With anyone going through difficult and painful rehabilitation, motivation is an important ingredient. Several of Lenny's friends who were traveling to or visiting California – Vermont pals like John Ruggiero, Mark Comolli and Jay Ward – planned to visit Lenny. Comolli was one of Lenny's best friends and, as the time for his visit approached, Lenny began to remember things they had done together, beginning his sentences with "Remember when me and Comolli ..." followed by some adventure they had shared. Lenny and Ruggiero had played basketball together and the two loved playing practical jokes on one another. When Lenny went up for varsity, Ruggiero told him he had to wear a suit and tie to games and Lenny believed him!

It was as Lenny progressed in his physical therapy that he began to remember his friends' arrival dates and look forward to them, but at the same time he began to have a growing appreciation of how different he was than when he was their schoolmate. Lenny began to talk about his conflicted feelings, which in turn demonstrated that his mental capabilities and the sophistication of his thought processes were growing. Some days, he felt the depth of his limitations and the work he needed to do while other days the promise of pie or visits from old friends inspired him to only work harder. Beyond all that, Lenny was intrinsically smart enough to know that much of what he was doing in rehab was the kind of exercise that one would do with a much younger child and he sometimes resented being treated as "a little kid." It was a tough time.

Nonetheless, in the weeks that followed, the therapists worked on Lenny's strength and coordination, while his mother studied the methodology, taking notes and carefully observing what worked best and what didn't. As both Lenny and Emmie discovered, the skills he, like other head-injured people, needed to work on were ones we take for granted: developing an almost unconscious orientation to one's surroundings, to what's happening in the world; relearning or learning for the first time basic life skills like writing checks or keeping track of appointments; making a list of what you might want to buy at the grocery store and figuring out how much money you need to buy what you want.

A newspaper helped with orientation, even a TV for the news. Notebooks were very important. Write it down, make a list. Lenny hated them. He did not want to write in a notebook. He resisted doing the exercises the therapists gave him, working on word recognition and matching. He'd had it with those word games. Emmie could understand his frustration at his slow progress, with having to do the same things over and over, and yet she knew intrinsically that repetition was the key to making pathways in the brain. She determined to bring fun into his life. Kathy and Gail would bring music to the ranch and dance with Lenny and the other clients during visiting hours. And on weekends there was the motel's pool and Pieloon.

Today, Emmie and Lenny agree that the time spent at Rancho Los Amigos was essential to where he is now, a 53-year-old man with a girlfriend, whose life is centered around helping those whose lives, like his, took a sudden, unforeseen turn, bringing them smack dab into a reality rife with frustration and opportunity. Indeed, Lenny's progress at Rancho was so positive that his therapists recommended he stay for another six weeks, concentrating on behavior and appropriateness. They thought that he could return to finish high school with just a little bit more work. When it was decided that he would remain, Kathy returned home and to school. But Emmie, knowing that she was probably the one doing the dishes and picking up at home, sent Kathy a little money every week. And when she had enough saved, Kathy wanted to buy a bicycle, a move that Len was absolutely dead set against, remembering Lenny's injuries. Emmie made sure she got the bike; one child's injury was not going to result in her other children not enjoying the pleasures and, yes, dangers of growing up.

Returning to Rutland after his time in California, Lenny told a reporter from the *Rutland Herald* in 1981, "When I had just barely come out of my coma and they told me I had a long road ahead of me just to walk again, I thought they were crazy. I thought I could just get up and walk away and I would be OK right away. But I soon saw that I was wrong. I knew it was going to be a long road for me. But right now I feel as positive about my future as I ever have. And much of that is due to the therapy I received in California."

Many of the skills and coping mechanisms he learned there have remained with him all these years later and in ways that the family was not yet ready to imagine became useful to others. Kathy, for example, has an autistic daughter with whom she uses some of the techniques she observed therapists use at the ranch. Clearly, she was a natural. Says Emmie, "She's very capable. She had early training."

Gail Austin was also deeply affected by her time spent with Lenny and at Rancho Los Amigos. She says she became a nurse because she became so fascinated with and impressed by the benefits that good nursing care could bring to a person's life.

When Lenny was ready to leave Rancho, the therapists made a discharge plan for those working with him back home. He would continue to work with Jim Kelley and others on his physical therapy, memory and other skills at home. By now, he was walking fairly well, although he had a bit of an awkward gait and his left arm remained positioned at an odd angle. Nonetheless, there were few people who had looked at his brain scan all those months previously who thought Lenny would ever walk again, not to mention do so as well as he had.

The discharge plan from Rancho Los Amigos had also made recommendations necessary for Lenny to return to high school to finish his interrupted senior year. Again, serendipity was with the Burkes.

Back home, a local man, Ron Savage, had returned to Rutland after earning his doctorate in learning and reading disorders from Boston University. He had previously received a master's degree in special education from Goddard College located in Plainfield, Vermont, and had a bachelor's degree in special education, from the Rutland, Vermont-based College of St. Joseph, graduating from all three summa cum laude. While he was getting his education, Savage worked with the Rutland school system as a learning disabilities and reading specialist and founded a summer learning clinic at the College of St. Joseph.

Like nearly everyone else in town, Savage knew Lenny's story and responded emotionally when Emmie contacted him to work with Lenny. "I was both excited and intimidated by the request. What do I know about traumatic brain injury? What therapies will work for Lenny? What if I really mess up and make things worse?" he asked himself. As it turned out, Savage's education had provided him with the skills that Lenny most needed at that time. There were people both at home and at MSJ who

Brain Injury Statistics

The following information is taken from the "Coma Guide for Caregivers" from the Delaware Health and Social Services of the Division of Services for Aging and Adults with Physical Disabilities, and is republished here with their express consent.

51% - Motor Vehicle Accidents
21% - Falls
12% - Assaults and Violence
10% - Sports and Recreation
6% - Other

A survivor of a severe brain injury faces 5 to 10 years of intensive services and rehabilitation.

The costs of a severe brain injury often exceed $4 million.

A majority of head injury survivors are under the age 30.

Two-thirds of those who survive will live a normal span of life, but will require life long services such as vocational rehabilitation and physical therapy.

A person does not need to be knocked out or lose consciousness to have sustained a traumatic brain injury.

A person does not need to strike his or her head to sustain traumatic brain injury (eg., whiplash, shaken baby syndrome).

Even mild traumatic brain injuries can cause cognitive impairments serious enough to impact a person's ability to enjoy life and to be able to work and earn a living.

People who sustain a brain injury are three times as likely to sustain a (second) brain injury.

Those who sustain a second brain injury are eight times as likely to sustain a (third) brain injury.

About 75 percent of all bicyclists who die each year die of head injuries.

85 percent of head injuries in bicycle accidents can be prevented by wearing a helmet.

Males between the ages of 14 and 24 have the highest rate of injury.

Males are almost twice as likely to suffer serious brain injuries than females.

Brain injuries kill more Americans under the age of 34 than all diseases combined.

Child abuse is the cause of 64 percent of all infant head injuries.

Approximately 1 in 500 school-age children each year receive a head injury severe enough to be hospitalized.

"After 25 years, I have come to believe that the only disability that human beings really suffer from is loneliness."

—The Rev. Richard Marceau

The Effects of Brain Injury

From The US Centers for Disease Control and Prevention

Brain injuries affect each person differently. Depending on the type of brain injury, the area of the brain affected and the extent of the injury, the effect of brain injury will vary from person to person. A person with a brain injury does not necessarily show all of the effects described below.

Coma:

When a brain injury is very severe, a person may slip into a state of coma. When someone is in a coma they are unconscious and although they may look as though they are asleep, they cannot be woken up. Someone in a coma is not able to respond, or speak or follow commands such as "open your eyes" or "squeeze my hand." They will not be able to move but may have some reflex muscle jerks or twitches.

A person can be in a coma for hours, days or several weeks, or longer. Coming out of a coma happens gradually and slowly, so at first they will drift in and out of coma. Nobody can predict how well they will come out of a coma because it depends on where in the brain the injury has occurred and the severity of the injury, amongst other factors. A person may come out of a coma with a combination of physical, cognitive and psychological difficulties that need special attention.

If the brain is so badly damaged the body needs to rest to allow the brain to heal, doctors will sometimes deliberately put someone in a coma, called a drug-induced coma. A drug-induced coma or controlled coma allows the body to switch off and focus on the healing process. Some people continue to show only very basic responses and will move from a coma into a minimally conscious state; others may recover quite well.

People often wonder if someone in a coma can hear or feel. And although it is impossible to know (because those who come out of a coma do not remember what it was like) it is recommended that we speak with and act around them as if they can hear, feel and understand.

Minimally Responsive State / Minimally Conscious State:

This term is used when a person is no longer in a coma and is more aware of themself or others around them. They can open their eyes, have a sleep-and-wake cycle and are able to respond with some movement such as blinking, but this is inconsistent or minimal. They sometimes appear to be tracking (following someone or something with their eyes). Someone can remain in a minimally conscious state for a very long time and may never come out of it, which means they will need a permanent high level of care.

Post-Traumatic Amnesia:

Post–traumatic amnesia (PTA) is a phase people go through following a significant brain injury, when they are confused, disoriented and have trouble with their memory. They may not be able to recall their date of birth, or may not know where they are or what has happened. When left alone they could be at risk of wandering and may be unable to find their way home or they may do risky things like leave on the oven in the kitchen.

People in PTA will be tested on a daily basis with a test called the Westmead PTA scale. This test has 12 questions, some concerning orientation such as "what day is it?" or "what year is it?"; other questions assess memory such as remembering objects or faces. This test is repeated each day and a score of one point is given for every correct answer. A person is considered to be emerging from PTA when their scores go up but they have to score 12 out of 12 three times in a row to be considered out of PTA.

Sometimes it is possible for someone to be oriented but still get the memory component of the test wrong, which tells us that he or she is not able to lay down new memories. Although most people come out of PTA eventually there is no set time for this because each person is different and each head injury heals at a different rate. Some people are in PTA for a few days or weeks; others for much longer.

Depending on the affected area of the brain and the severity of injury, a person may experience physical effects such as:

- Weakness of one or more limbs. In some cases, a person may experience paralysis or the inability to move one side of their body, which is called hemiplegia. Having difficulty moving both upper and lower limbs is called a quadriparesis.
- Difficulty with coordination or precise, fine-tuned movements.
- Difficulty with balance, for example being unable to sit unsupported, stand up without help or walk without help. Sometimes losing balance means that the person is at a risk of falls and may need a walking aid.
- Difficulty with high or low muscle tone, or with 'switching-on or switching-off' muscles. When there is a problem with low muscle tone, a person may have difficulty using a limb; for example a low-toned arm may hang lifeless next to the body and cannot be used for reaching or supporting. When there is a problem with high tone, a person may not be able to use a limb properly because the muscles tighten up, pulling their arm or leg into awkward and maybe painful positions. People with very high muscle tone may develop a condition called spasticity, which causes muscles to seize up, be resistant to stretching and to cause stiffness in the limb. Spasticity goes hand in hand with exaggerated reflexes and spasm, or violent and painful muscle jerks.
- Difficulty with swallowing, speech or vision.
- Difficulty with sensation or feeling in one or more parts of the body, for example not being aware where the arm is without looking or having difficulty feeling touch, pressure, hot or cold.
- Having difficulty with toileting - lacking the feeling to control bladder or bowels.
- High levels of fatigue, which is different from being tired after a long day's work. This fatigue is more of a mental fatigue, making the person unable to concentrate or participate because the brain shuts down.

Cognitive effects of brain injury may include:

- Poor memory, especially short-term memory. Memory problems may include the inability to lay down new memories and/or retrieve them when they are needed.
- Poor reasoning skills - not being able to weigh up several options and choose the best option. Being unable to make choices.
- Poor problem solving skills - unable to analyze a problem and find solutions to solve that problem.

- Poor attention span - not able to divide attention or not able to concentrate on something. Being easily distracted.
- Poor safety awareness or insight into their limitations.
- Poor judgement - not seeing the consequences of a chosen behavior.
- Poor initiation - requiring prompting to start or complete tasks or activities.

Psychological effects of brain injury may include:

- Inappropriate behavior – being unable to judge right from wrong such as making inappropriate comments or showing inappropriate behaviors. This may include inappropriate sexual behavior such as exposing themself in public, or touching other people inappropriately or making sexual inappropriate remarks. Other inappropriate behaviors may be interrupting other people's conversations, making bad jokes or rude or socially unacceptable comments or inappropriate laughter. Demonstrating these behaviors may be embarrassing for family and friends and may cause a person to become isolated.
- Violent and aggressive behavior – being unable to control emotions, resulting in verbal or physical aggressive behavior such as swearing, shouting, hitting out, biting, spitting, punching or throwing objects.
- Emotional disregulation - being unable to control emotions such as happiness and showing excessive laughter or giggling, or showing excessive sorrow such as crying.
- Being more at risk of being depressed, paranoid, anxious, or showing signs of being disconnected from reality.
- Difficulty with detecting others' emotions; for example not noticing that someone close to them is upset or angry, or not showing interest in other people's emotions or being able to adapt their behavior to other people's emotions. This detachment from other people's emotions can cause a lot of stress and disappointment in relationships. It may change someone's relationship completely and may cause rifts in partnerships.

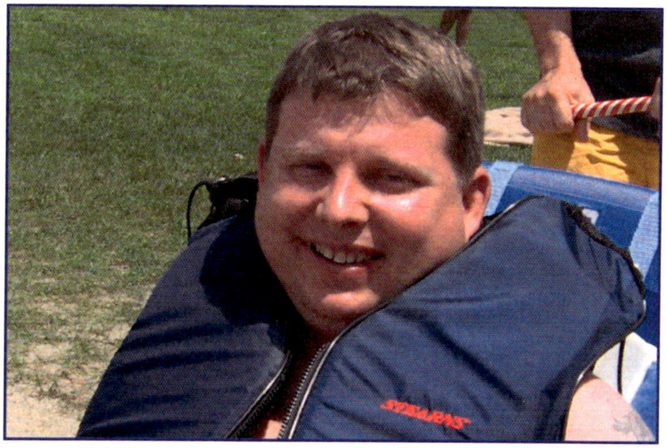

Christopher Patrick Russell enjoys an outing at Elfin Lake in Wallingford.

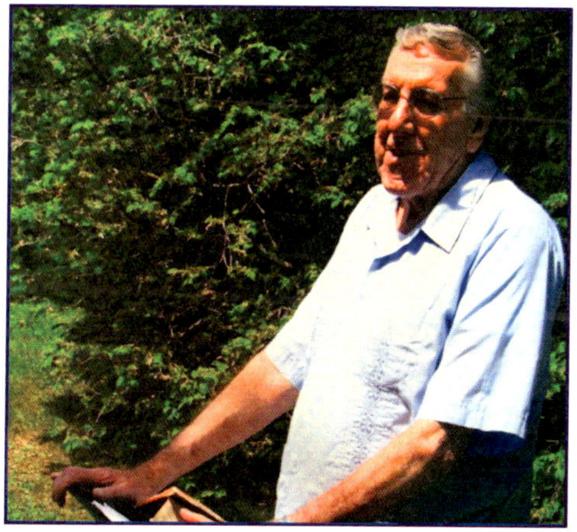

The Rev. Richard Marceau

HIS Independence Project, Inc.

NEWSLETTER

SUMMER 1986 "HELP MAKE LIFE AFTER HEAD INJURY BETTER IN VERMONT"

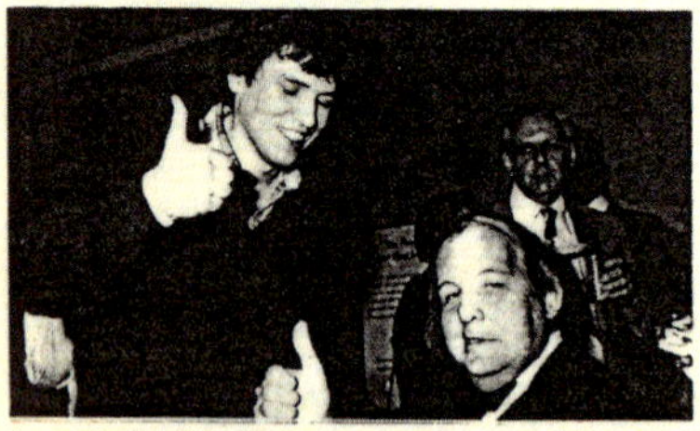

Thumbs up for the convention!

Lenny Burke of the Vermont Head Injury Foundation and James Brady, press secretary to the President, signal "thumbs up" to indicate the success of the NHIF's first annual convention. (More photos on page 8.)

CONVENTION/BOARD MEETING SCORES A HIT!

Over 300 members of the NHIF and their guests gathered in Washington, D.C. April 16-19 to convene the Foundation's first annual convention/ Board meeting, "Building for the Future." As the participants came together for workshops, panel discussions and informal meetings, it became readily apparent that this gathering of head injury survivors, family members and professionals was designed for success.

A Day of Advocacy

The first day of the convention was devoted to advocacy as members of the NHIF attended workshops in the morning (see accompanying story) and kept previously made appointments with their respective legislators in the afternoon. Lunch was held in the Russell Building Caucus Room as Senators John C. Danforth (R-MO) and Edward M. Kennedy (D-MA) were honored for their legislative efforts on behalf of head injured persons. John A. Doyle, executive director of the National Association of Rehabilitation Facilities (NARF) was the afternoon guest speaker.

NATIONAL HEAD INJURY FOUNDATION (NHIF)

This newsletter contains articles from the NHIF Spring 1986 Newsletter - Vol. 6, no. 1 and is reprinted with their permission

The first day's activities were capped off by a reception held in honor of James Brady, press secretary to the President. Attended by guests from the Senate and the House of Representatives as well as convention attendees, the reception provided all with the opportunity to meet and chat with Mr. Brady.

During the reception, members were able to preview the newest NHIF public service announcement (PSA) featuring Mr. Brady as spokesperson for the Foundation. This PSA, produced with the assistance of the public relations firm Needham, Porter, Novelli of Washington, D.C., will be released in the fall in conjunction with National Head Injury Awareness Month, and we are most grateful to Mr. Brady for his willingness to speak out on behalf of head injury survivors around the country.

Exhibits Highlight Second Day

Presentations, workshops and evening exhibits highlighted the second day of the convention as members were able to interact with speakers and experts in the field of head injury on topics that included, among others, developing community based residential programs, building a funding base and developing OSERS state agency agreements.

Morning sessions opened with presentations by Thomas Gustafson, Ph.D., director, Div. of Medicaid and Long Term Care Policy, Health Care Finan-

Continued on page 6

NHIF reprint

ADVOCACY ON THE HILL

The major reason for holding the first annual NHIF convention in Washington, D.C. was to bring our membership to the attention of the members of Congress who create the entitlement and eligibility legislation that affects every aspect of services for head injured people.

The morning was spent listening to panel discussions chaired by Jack Duncan, Esq., NHIF governmental affairs advisor, as he reviewed issues that are of great importance to head injured persons. Mr. Duncan was most emphatic in his assertion that NHIF advocacy efforts have and will continue to play a critical role in the realization of services for those who have survived head injuries.

Panel members, which included David Esquith, minority legislative associate, House Subcommittee on Select Education; Christine Ferguson, legislative assistant to Senator John Chaffee; Gary Garwood, staff director, House Subcommittee on Select Education; Judy Wagner, legislative assistant to Senator Paul Simon; and Sally Yozell, minority professional staff member, Senate Subcommittee on the Handicapped, summarized in some detail the individual bills currently under discussion in Congress. This discussion made it quite apparent that the first order of business was to ensure the reauthorization of the Rehabilitation Act of 1973 and of PL 94-142, the Education of the Handicapped Act.

In addition, there was a discussion of Senator Chaffee's bill, the Community and Family Living Amendment of 1985, which amends Title XIX of the Social Security Act to fund severely disabled individuals to receive community and residential placement services, and of the Bartlett Bill, section 1619 of the Social Security Bill, which stresses supportive work for the severely disabled without the loss of Medicaid benefits.

The morning ended with presentations by Paul Marchand, director, Governmental Affairs of the Association for Retarded Citizens, and chairperson

Continued on page 5

NHIF reprint

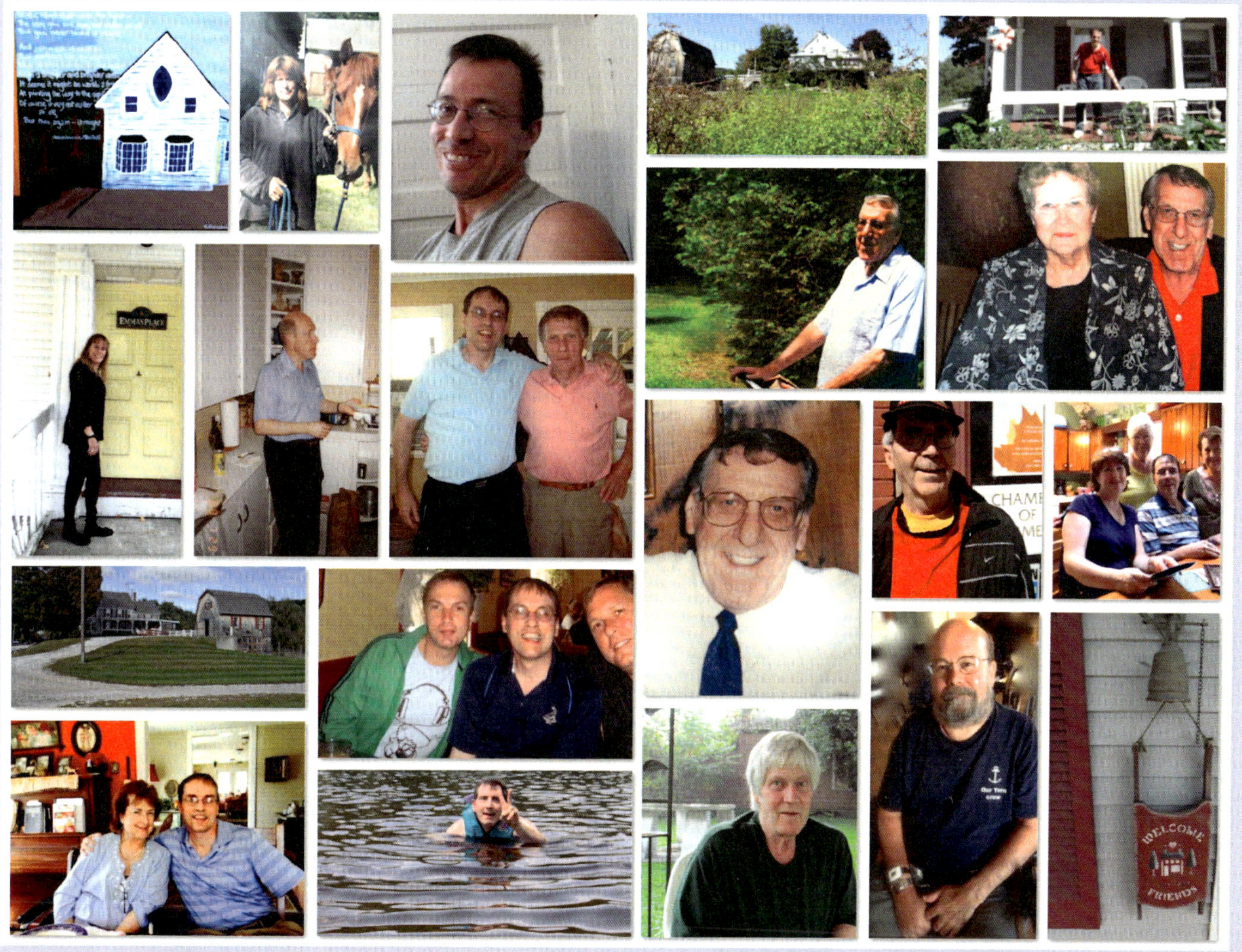

> "Thoughts are seeds . . . The thoughts I give time and space to in my mind are going to produce outcomes."
>
> *–The Rev. Richard Marceau*

could help him with his physical therapy. What Lenny needed were readiness skills so that he could reintegrate into a school where he'd once been "like a god," and earn his diploma, ideally in the fall of 1980. Savage immediately set out to find educators trained to work with someone like Lenny. Enter Tricia Mulholland, one of Savage's students who specialized in cognitive remediation, and Karlene Foy Marro, another graduate student at the College of St. Joseph's learning clinic, who helped develop learning strategies that would become essential to Lenny's growth and maturity. The two women worked to provide Lenny with tools to improve his attention span and concentration, supplemented with strategies to monitor his own behavior and appropriateness.

Savage was there to reinforce these therapists, instinctively understanding that the damage to Lenny's brain had altered Lenny's natural reticence. He talked to Lenny about using the skills he had honed on the basketball court and golf range – patience, timing and consideration – in daily life. Unlike so many other therapists, Savage had seen Lenny on the court; he knew those skills were there, if damaged, and he sought to bring them out and then reinforce them. Recalls Savage, "I remember bringing Lenny over to my house because my sons thought he was the 'best basketball teacher in the world.' My young sons did not care about Lenny's brain injury; for them it did not even exist. What existed was Lenny's joy in helping them make a jump shot or cross dribble between their legs."

The two worked closely over the summer to prepare Lenny for Mount St. Joseph Academy. He would be a senior alongside brother Kevin. Throughout that summer, as Savage and Marro worked closely with Lenny, they were also working hand and hand with Emmie, sharing what they knew about literal and inferential comprehension, sharing methods for teaching social and emotional development, and something called "over learning," that is teaching some skill, then reinforcing it again and again to compensate for memory problems. Together, the three developed a 16-page case study with recommendations to be utilized in creating a lesson plan for Lenny's final year of high school. Emmie's job would be to reinforce what he had learned in school as part of his homework and Marro's job was to coordinate between his teachers to help keep him on track.

At the same time, Lenny worked with Dr. William Frey, a psychotherapist whose job it was to help Lenny relearn how to read social prompts and act more appropriate for his age. For Frey, who'd not worked with a person who had sustained a traumatic brain injury before, the sessions were instructive. He came to see that much of what he'd been taught or had assumed about TBI was only partially true. As he helped Lenny navigate through the emotional landscape of adolescence, Lenny was teaching him that the brain could relearn.

Lenny's progress may have been slower than he wanted but there was progress. He regained the ability to write. His first letter was to Chris Cooper, a blind masseur at the Cortina Inn who gave Lenny a massage twice a week in an attempt to relax muscles still over-restricted from his injury. In the letter, Lenny wrote, "The massage takes him 45 minutes to an hour. After he's done, he says: 'Lenny, stand up and tell me how you feel.' I say, 'Chris, have you ever been in heaven?'" Lenny may have been slowed down but he hadn't lost his sense of humor.

But there were struggles as well. Lenny found it hard to concentrate in class and harder still to sit still. Even with all the work that had been done on self-control, he was very spontaneous and would talk out of turn, sometimes inappropriately. After all, he was a teenager full of teenage hormones back in the company of young people – translate girls – his own age. Due to the head injury, he sometimes forgot to censor his thoughts and reactions. And because of his lessened attention span, he couldn't sit through a whole football or basketball game. Instead, someone in the family, often Kevin or Michael, would take him for just the end of a game. Lenny loved that. But there's no question that it was a tough year for Lenny, Michael and Kevin. After all, this was Kevin's senior year and here was Lenny, his hero, back in school a different person than the one he'd always looked up to. Michael had had to face the reality that Lenny couldn't be fixed into the old Lenny when he returned from Rancho Los Amigos. Still, that acceptance was a lot different from having your brother acting odd or inappropriate when you are just a freshman in high school.

Nonetheless, Michael says, "Honestly. I've never resented Lenny. I never experienced jealousy for him. I always felt supported by him." He also notes that his mother's concentration on Lenny allowed him and Kevin to develop self-reliance at an early age along with the knowledge that life can change in a second. Of course, knowledge of one's vulnerability at an early age can trigger both good and bad behaviors. One result was some unhealthy behavior on both Kevin and Michael's parts from their late teens into their twenties. Both struggled with substance abuse and, perhaps as a result, both have chosen to remain sober for nearly 25 years.

Perhaps as important, Michael says the sudden change in Lenny's stature, so shocking and freeing at the same time, and Lenny's ability to persevere through it all, remaining cheerful despite so many challenges, gave him the strength to make difficult decisions at an early age.

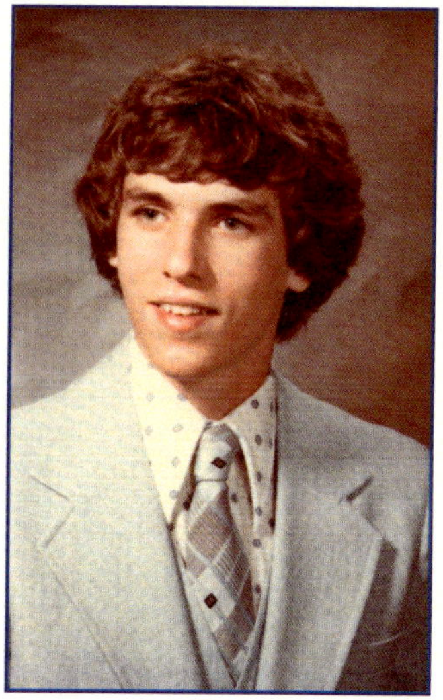

Lenny's graduation photo.

And despite the obstacles, Lenny graduated as planned. In an article published in the *Rutland Herald* around the time of his graduation, Lenny told a reporter, "I didn't like it when I had to ask for help, especially from my brothers and sister. It bothered me and it bothered them, because they had always looked up to me. But we got over that and they've been with me every step of the way." In what now seems prophetic, he told the reporter that he might like to be a "physical therapist. So many of them have helped me and I would like to do the same. I probably know more about rehabilitation than anyone, and I'd like to share it."

The article ended with this quote from Lenny: "I can remember the feeling I used to have when I took my best shot, the baseline jumper. I always had this strong feeling that I could never miss, and even when I did miss, I felt that it was just a fluke and I would hit it the next time. I think in the last few months I've started to get that same kind of faith in myself back. There was a time when I was trying to say that I couldn't make it back, but now I know I just have to transfer that faith to the things that I will do in my new life."

Lenny's senior year was tough on Marro, too. Lenny knew MSJ backwards and forwards – the school's layout was safe and secure in his long-term

Sally Carleton: But Were They Ever Wrong!

When Sally Carleton hosts her "Horse Ladies Lunch Club," she doesn't talk about her brain injury. She talks about her favorite subjects: riding, caring for and just plain loving horses. Her horse Angus, now 20, a big, handsome Belgian workhorse and Morgan cross, is, like her, Vermont-born and Vermont-independent.

That's why it thrills her to remember that doctors told her not just that she would never ride again but that she would not recover from the brain injury she sustained when she had an aneurism while driving on Dorr Drive in Rutland on Sept. 19, 1999, and slammed into a house at 40 mph.

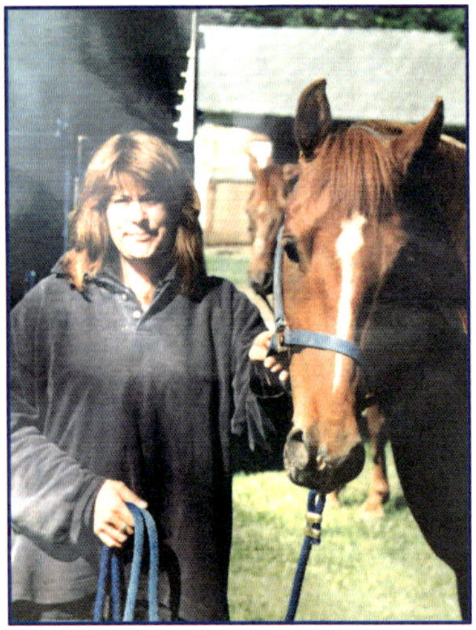

"They said I would have issues with my brain and balance forever, that I would be tremendously mindfully disabled," she recalls. "Boy, were they ever wrong."

"They didn't know me and they didn't know my husband," she says of the musician and filmmaker Duane Carleton. "He was there every day. He'd come to see me at 2:30 in the morning if he had to, driving late to the hospital after a gig and he'd stay with me every night, night after night. Without fail."

It's not that Carleton – a woman with a deep, soulful singing voice who grew up on a Vermont farm – does not continue to struggle with limitations that resulted from the aneurism and resulting brain injury. But she has three major things going for her: the support of her husband; her responsibilities working at Lenny Burke's Farm; and the ability to enjoy the activities that have always given her life meaning: riding her horses and caring for her dog, painting signs, being out in nature, and music.

Carleton had to learn to walk and talk again during her rehabilitation at Rutland Hospital. She also benefitted from sessions with Dr. William Frey, a now-retired psychotherapist who developed a specialty in working with people who had sustained traumatic brain injuries and their families after he worked with Lenny Burke and his family.

Carleton said that work was essential for her and her husband. "It was a difficult time and he sailed us through it. It was so hard. I was a woman who rode horses and motorcycles, who lived life at full tilt. I had to be convinced I was not the super-hot two-day overnight horse rider I used to be but that the things I loved could be had, just at a different level. I learned to start thinking smarter in how to approach life.

"I'm lucky but it took me a while to see that. I had to say to myself, 'You've got a healthy environment. Your husband loves you.' I figured out I am a little disabled. I don't have the stamina I once had; I get tired and have a little weakness on the right side. Okay, so I'm not as good as I was but I'm okay," she says.

"But most of all, I gained a lot of humility from this injury. It's only happened because of working at Lenny Burke's Farm. I've seen more than a handful of people who had a similar injury and didn't make it half the way back. I'm able to care for myself. When I need help, I can say I need help. And I know it will be there."

Governor's Awards to Lenny Burke Farm, Its Founder and Staff

Reverend Richard Marceau, Professional of the Year, 1997

Emma Burke, Professional of the Year, 1999

Kevin Burke, Professional of the Year, 2000

Hugh Barclay, Professional of the Year, 2006

Kathy Chandler, Caregiver of the Year, 2007

Mary Pearce, Caregiver of the Year, 2008

Barbara Barron-Rolfe, Caregiver of the Year, 2001

Duane Carleton, Caregiver of Year, 2000

Lenny Burke's Farm, Employer of the Year, 2010

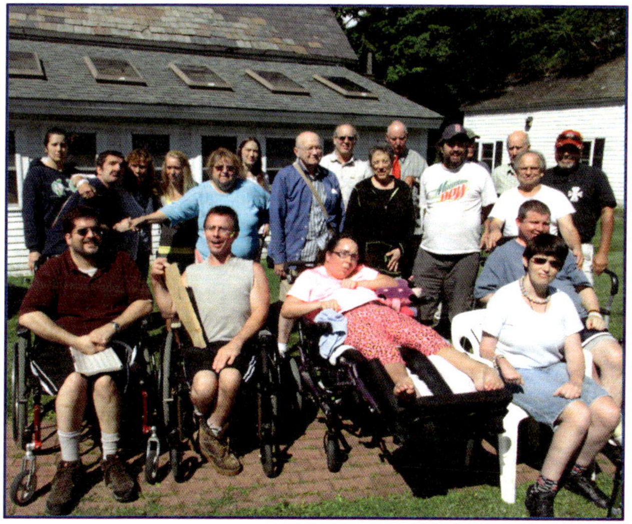

The Possibility of Magic

By Sherry Howarth

If you have had the great good fortune of knowing Lenny Burke before one game on the Mount Saint Joseph basketball court rocked his world and the community he had shone so brightly in, I wager you are smiling inside and out to learn more of his remarkable story.

I was a senior at Mill River Union High School in North Clarendon, just a few miles from MSJ at the time he was injured, working hard with my classmates to win the coveted Regional One Act Play Festival honors.

We had chosen an extremely emotive play, "The Trial of the Catonsville Nine" by the Berrigan Brothers about their Vietnam protest experience. Mighty fine Stage 40/theatre director and English teacher Peter Marsh made some wonder happen with a few earnest high school kids.

Our guidance counselor, Art Crandall, who'd previously worked at MSJ, had been very much a part of the rehearsals, but one late Tuesday night in January he hadn't slipped in the back to hang out in the lighting booth.

Then, when we were nearly done with rehearsal, Crandall hit both the auditorium main doors with everything he had, his face drained of color as the sound of the doors hitting the back wall reverberated through the empty auditorium.

His news rocked our world, too, but immediately Marsh announced we would pause working on our one-act play to present several benefit performances to help raise money for Lenny. We could be useful.

Now, all these years later, I've had the privilege of working for Lenny for about 12 years. I consider him my hero.

Adds David Hardy, my husband, who has worked at the farm for a decade now, "All shifts have the possibility of magic."

memory – and he'd often just get up and leave a class to wander the halls. In the 1981 yearbook under his name, you'll find this question, "Has anyone seen Lenny?" attributed to Marro whose supervision he found rather clever ways to circumvent.

That said, Marro – who like Savage had never worked with a person with a severe brain injury before Lenny and was initially intimidated by "the magnitude of the task" – says that her work with Lenny "became personally and professionally the most rewarding learning experience of my life." Like so many people who became involved in the Lenny Burke story, Marro continued as a resource, traveling with Lenny and Emmie to the Woodrow Wilson Rehabilitation Center in Fisherville, Virginia, in the summer of 1981 after Lenny's graduation. She wanted to help facilitate Lenny's orientation to the facility, sharing with them what she knew of his responses and needs. That fall, Lenny attended the center for a few months but found the separation from his family difficult. Beyond that, he'd had it with the routine of the same old exercises. As he told his family, it was time to get on with life, a decision that came just as a new chapter in the story was unfolding.

That unfolding was a joint realization between Emmie, Rev, Ron Savage, Marion Austin, Bill Frey, and others in the community who had either experienced a traumatic brain injury or knew someone who had that something had to be done about the lack of support services in Vermont. Emmie had been urged by the therapists at Rancho Los Amigos to form a national or state organization; working on the state level seemed the best way to proceed. She still recalls a life-changing conversation she and Savage had about this time. "Ron and I were talking about the fact that we didn't have any of the services that were needed in Vermont and he said, 'We are waiting for someone who will do it, but it's us.'"

They named their organization H.I.S., short for Head Injury/Stroke Independence Project. Its articles of incorporation spell out the organization's philosophy: to provide "coordination of services to traumatically brain-injured or stroke individuals within their home environment and places of employment or training and provide direct, cognitive, effective training to such individuals and undertake to train the individual's family." The idea of home-based therapy grew out of the organizers' understanding that what people with severe brain injuries needed most was "to gain independence and participate as fully as possible in their local communities … using available resources." In this, Emmie and her cohorts were working from practical experience, establishing manageable goals that recognized each individual's challenges and strengths and the resources available to them. That practical approach was twinned with the philosophy that it is always better to look at what a person can do and build from there rather than concentrate on what a person cannot do.

Emmie worked closely with Marilyn Spivak, a woman whose story echoed that of the Burke family. In 1974, like Emmie, Spivak was a wife and mother

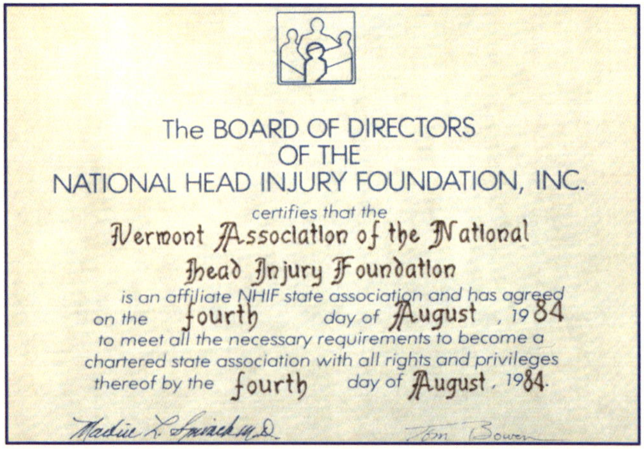
The BOARD OF DIRECTORS
OF THE
NATIONAL HEAD INJURY FOUNDATION, INC.
certifies that the
Vermont Association of the National
Head Injury Foundation
is an affiliate NHIF state association and has agreed
on the fourth day of August, 1984
to meet all the necessary requirements to become a
chartered state association with all rights and privileges
thereof by the fourth day of August, 1984.

whose life took a dramatic turn when her youngest daughter Deborah sustained a traumatic brain injury in a motor vehicle accident, resulting in a prolonged coma and lifelong disability. (The family suffered another tragedy the following year when their son Jon was killed in a motorcycle accident.)

After five years of frustration trying to find an appropriate rehabilitation program for her daughter, she and her husband Martin worked with other families and professionals to form the National Head Injury Foundation (now the Brain Injury Association of America.) From the beginning, H.I.S has had a strong relationship with the national organization – Emmie was the 17th person to join the organization that now has thousands of members and affiliates; the relationship continues to today.

Again, local supporters came to Emmie's aid, people like attorney John Crowley, a neighbor and friend who helped with the complex paperwork to create a nonprofit organization. And there was Thomas Trombetta, a local man who had sustained a spinal cord injury playing in a jump house with his children. The late Katherine Sivret, a good friend with three sons, the youngest of whom had died of leukemia, offered her services as did the late Lloyd Kelley, a longtime educator whose son had died from a head injury after a car accident. Elizabeth Walter, a local woman who worked at a nursing home, came aboard; she had a special interest in helping people whose cognitive abilities had been impaired by head injury or stroke. And there was Rev, of course.

In reading the notes from the group's early meetings and reports of its activities, it's clear that what these people had in common was not just a personal interest in traumatic brain injuries, but more important a deep understanding of something Rev was fond of repeating. It was his take on an Aldous

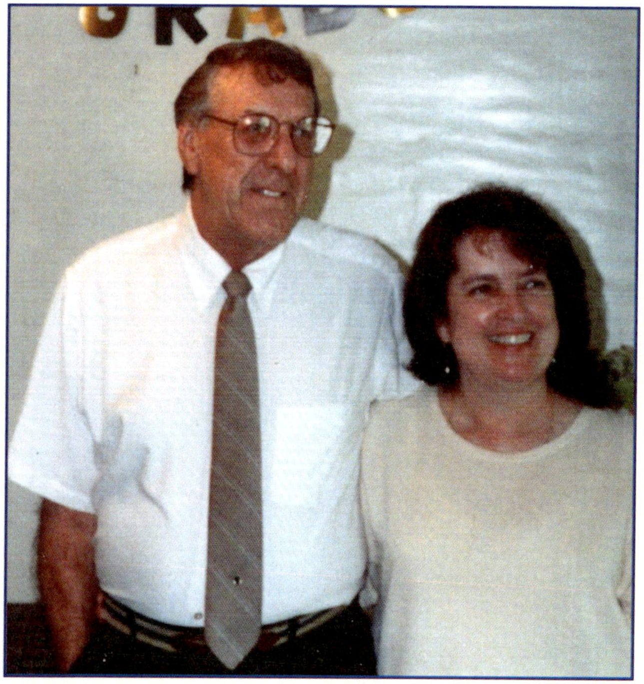

Emmie and Rev in the early days of H.I.S.

Huxley mantra: "Experience is not what happens to a man; it is what a man does with what happens to him." Rev's version: "It's not what happens to us that makes a difference … It's how we choose to respond to it that makes all the difference." For Rev, that word "choose" had superpower.

Within weeks of the organization's founding, Emmie and Ron Savage found themselves traveling Vermont to provide support services to families whose children had sustained head injuries and visiting hospitals and nursing homes where heartbreaking stories were unfolding. Much of

Tim's Story: It's Not the End of the Road Montessori and Family Connections

By Paula Monahan
(Editor's note: This story from a woman not connected to Lenny Burke's Farm shows yet another way in which instinct, courage and experimentation worked together to help an individual who had sustained three traumatic brain injuries.)

In the year 2000 my husband Tim suffered the first of three insults to his brain.

It was January. We packed our van for a winter vacation to Florida and planned to leave the next morning. We were watching a PBS documentary of George Washington when Tim excused himself, put the television on pause and headed to the bathroom. All of a sudden I heard banging, as if he were bouncing off the walls. He came lurching into the family room and fell on the couch. His face was becoming purple. I dialed 911. He was rushed to the hospital where he was operated on for a ruptured aortic aneurysm or Triple A as it was referred to from then on.

He was transferred to Mass General and eventually to Spaulding Rehab where we began the long journey back. Various therapists worked with him each day, as did I. I continued my daily practice of reading to him, singing to him, playing imaginary rounds of golf with him. I also brought in games I had used with my kindergarten students. Everything came together and after months of hospital and rehab, we were able to go home.

The second insult came months later.

Tim experienced an embolic stroke (a clot thrown by the heart). The stroke did incredible damage to Tim's brain. One of the intensive care doctors showed me just how much of Tim's brain was blown away. He said, "I am so sorry." I countered with, "Don't be. You don't know my husband." By that, I meant that he was a can do kind of guy. There wasn't anything he wouldn't tackle.

Eventually, we made it to rehab. Tim had aphasia because the stroke hit his language center. He wasn't able to use his arm or leg on his right side and therapists once again worked with him. Their time was limited, so it was up to me to make the most of his day.

I started out at the very beginning with my European Montessori training. He had to relearn everything. I used Montessori's Three Period lesson to teach. He progressed. I brought in children's games that promote learning (e.g. memory, concentration, perceptual tasks). I also brought in paints and we painted (something he never would have attempted prior to this!).

He improved slowly and eventually he came home.

He still needed a lot of help walking with his leg in a full-length cast. The therapist worked three times a week. A friend and I took him to a local school gym and worked on helping him move. We videotaped his small victories.

I brought him to Dr. Lee Schwam in Boston. He asked Tim if he wanted to walk again. Tim nodded vigorously and attempted a garbled "Yes!" The doctor said, "Then you will." The first time he moved that leg, we felt we had landed on the moon!

We took him out to try his beloved game of golf. He was propped up in a cart between two women. We would stand him at his ball, put a club in his hand and he connected!

The third insult to Tim's brain came when he catapulted himself out of his automatic chair, hit his head on his desk and had a brain bleed.

By now we knew the drill: neuro intensive care, the hospital floor, rehab and home. Therapists still came. I would roll him on to a standing table, crank him up and watch him enjoy seeing the ships and boats going up and down the river.

He still grew connections, played games with us and experienced life. He was confined to a wheelchair at this point. He was included in all of our children's important moments: graduations, weddings and holidays.

Tim died August 31, 2005.

When elements of love, sharing experiences, come together, one can grow the neuro connections needed to recover. It was our family connections that helped Tim's brain recover.

Exposures to blasts are a leading cause of TBI among active duty military personnel in war zones.

Veterans' advocates believe that between 10 and 20 percent of Iraq veterans, or at least 150,000 and 300,000 service members have some level of TBI.

30 percent of soldiers admitted to Walter Reed Army Medical Center have been diagnosed as having had a TBI.

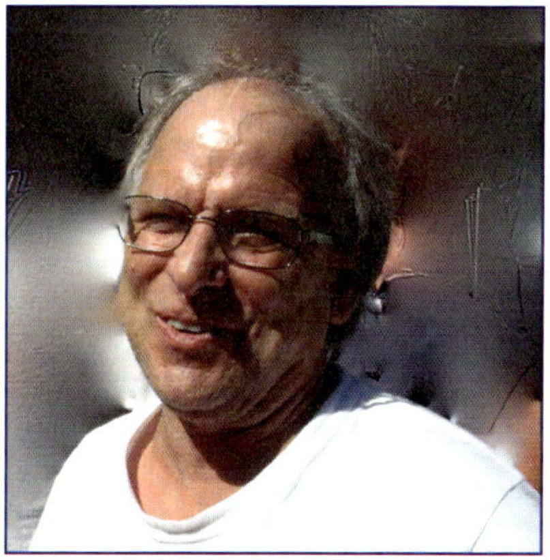

David Coffman enjoys writing songs and poems, painting flower pots and singing at Lenny Burke's Farm.

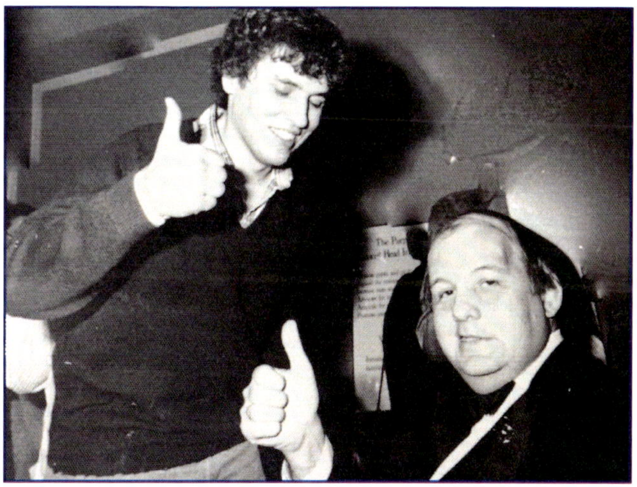

Percent Distributions of TBI-related Hospitalizations by Age Group and Injury Mechanism — United States, 2006–2010

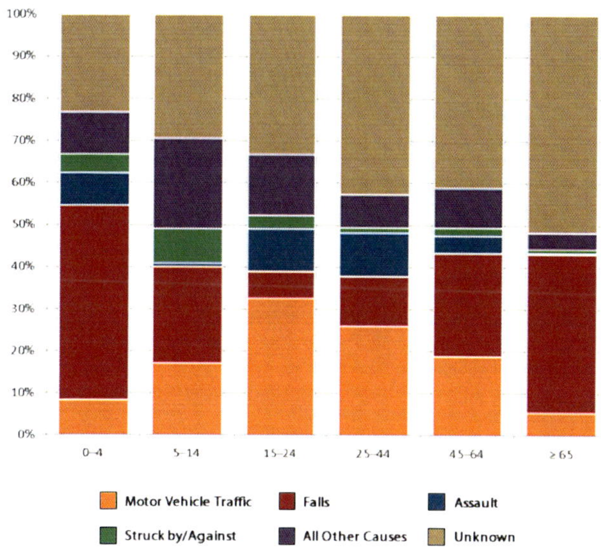

the work was being done on a volunteer basis. At the same time, Rev would lead meetings he called "serendipity gatherings" at different people's homes or at church. His question: What would you do if you could do anything you wanted? Emmie's answer one day was, "I would like to build a place large enough for lots of people with head injuries to live." Immediately, Elizabeth Walter, the friend who worked at a local nursing home, remembered that she had heard about a new state grant program that aimed to help people with disabilities stay in their own homes. Serendipity indeed.

Emmie set out to write a letter to the late Vermont Sen. Edgar May and others in charge of the state's nascent Independence Fund. Later, May told her what happened to that letter: The committee read it, noticed the lack of credentials and work history on the part of its author, and threw the letter into the wastebasket. Then the committee members read the rest of the applicants' letters. None of them appealed to the committee members. Finally, one of the members said something like, "Let's pull that letter out of the wastebasket about working with TBI." They did and decided to take a chance on this unproven woman with no statistics or budget to back up her dreams of creating a support system for people with head injuries and their caregivers. H.I.S. was awarded $35,000, which allowed Emmie and Savage to set up shop in a small office in downtown Rutland and start working with families directly in their homes. Beginning then, therapists at the newly established Center for Independent Learning started contacting Emmie or Rev or Ron Savage about people they heard about who were in nursing homes but didn't belong there or families struggling as they cared for a recovering family member at home.

H.I.S. also organized countless informational and support group meetings for the general public and offered free workshops on brain injury for educators, medical and service care professionals throughout Vermont. Efforts were made to create a Vermont chapter of the National Head Injury Foundation and in 1984 an organizational meeting toward that end was held at Castleton State College. Eventually, Emmie decided to concentrate her efforts to Vermont. Meanwhile, Savage was expanding his education in the treatment and prevention of head injuries and had become the president of the National Head Injury Educational Task Force on Children and Youth. America was just becoming aware of the national epidemic of head injuries, particularly among children injured in sports and in bicycle and motor vehicle accidents, and he was eager to be part of this new movement. He was among the first to speak nationally about the importance of protective helmets.

Many creative projects came out of these first few years of working together. Savage was instrumental in creating the first-ever workshop on the issue for special educators held in Boston in 1985. He helped write a manual for educators working with individuals with head injuries that subsequently became a book. He and Lenny traveled together as spokespersons for the National Head Injury Foundation, visited with legislators who sought information on the prevalence and treatment of head injuries, and at every opportunity promoted a positive, proactive approach to treatment. Their message echoed Rev's: it's not what people can't do; it's finding a way to help them live up to their greatest potential. At the same time, Emmie developed a support program for young people with developmental disabilities; these young people started their own business making greeting cards. Dr. Bernie Buteau, a Rutland dentist whose son had sustained a head injury, organized a marathon that served as a fundraiser for H.I.S. while also spreading the word that people with head injuries could be helped and that part of their recovery included paying special attention to their physical needs. Indeed, Buteau was the first dentist to write professionally about the importance of dental care after a traumatic brain injury, even when a patient is in a coma. He knew some of the medications used for seizure control take a beating on teeth and that the pressure of seizures, much like teeth-grinding, can cause myriad problems that often go undetected and, therefore, untreated.

The late Jeff Phelps, a popular DJ and teacher who had polio as a child, joined the group, as did special educator Gabi Rubins, physiatrist Dr. Johanna Ruess from the Medial Center of Vermont, and Bob Franzoni, a retired businessman who just happened to be baseball great Ted Williams' best friend. Williams became an honorary member of the H.I.S. board and supported the organization throughout his lifetime. The late Theresa Mulholland, a principal at Wallingford (VT) Elementary School who had been one of Savage's students who got interested in brain injuries, joined the board and acted as a conduit to many of the local schools. Countless workshops and training sessions were offered throughout Vermont as more and more people realized both the prevalence of head injuries as well as the need for early intervention and proactive therapy. All these received the attention of Vermont's Congressional delegation, which along with supporting the work H.I.S. was doing also began paying attention to the prevalence of brain injuries and the need for preventative legislation and funding for services.

In the first year alone, the organization had 50 inquiries for help and within four years had provided services to more than 500 families. Rev was an essential ingredient in this success as he was often called in to help grieving families who were struggling to understand how to care for family members coming home from a hospital. "Emmie," he'd say, "I've heard of this case you might want to look into." Or, "Emmie, let's take Lenny and go visit my new friend who's only 28 but living in a nursing home because they just don't know what to do with him."

Like Rev, Emmie and the other people in her network of friends and specialists were quite aware of the need for more. Many of the people they met were in danger of becoming homeless; families were being stretched beyond their means, patience and abilities caring for children, husbands and wives who had sustained a traumatic brain injury. Emmie thought back to the statement she'd made at Rev's serendipity gathering and began to envision that home where she and Lenny and perhaps some other family members might work together to improve the living conditions for these individuals. Indeed, just as Emmie had articulated the desire to create a home-based treatment center for people with traumatic brain injuries, Lenny began to understand that he had something to offer others in a similar condition. Thanks to the unusually focused attention he had received, he had progressed much further than any of the specialists had anticipated. While he still had problems with short-term memory, he had learned strategies for essentially putting important information into his long-term memory.

Perhaps as important, he'd developed a healthy sense of humor about his memory issues. He knew he could recall names and dates from the past better than some of those around him. And while his walk was somewhat awkward and his left arm impaired, he could share what he knew about basketball with others even if he'd lost that perfect shot. During these years, he worked as an assistant basketball coach at a host of local schools, an effort that continued until

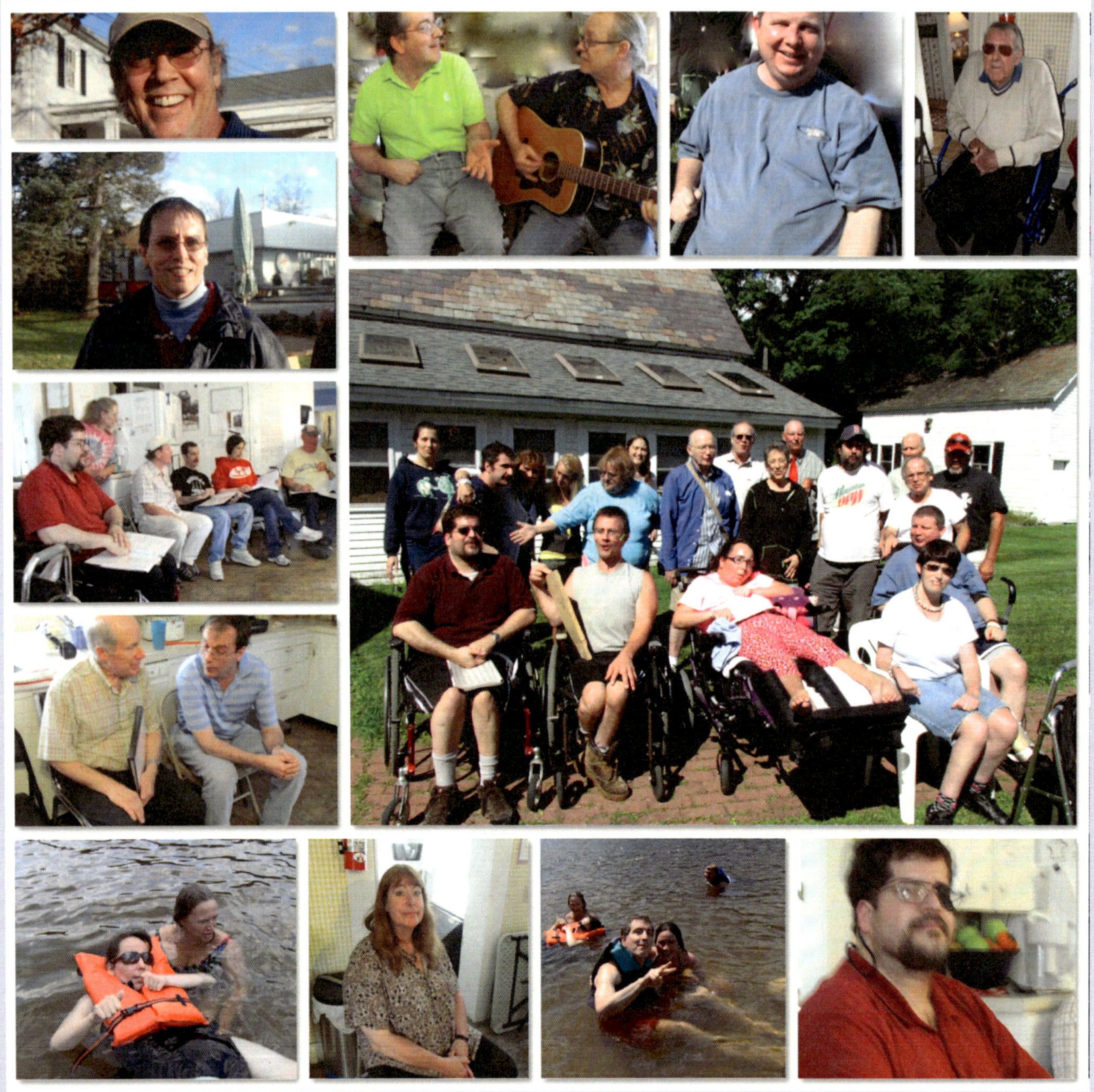

"If you come to a fork in the road, take it." —Yogi Berra

Hannah Bondioli: Another Ripple in the Pool

Hannah Bondioli says her big sister Emmie was always saving her life. Then, she'll add that it was Lenny who helped her save her own.

"Lenny was part of the catalyst that got me sober," she says. "The night he was hurt, my friend and neighbor Kim and her four little ones had moved into my house. Her husband, who was drunk, had shot a rifle through their bedroom wall into the living room where the children were pretending to camp in their sleeping bags. I didn't know what had happened to Lenny until later the next morning when Mother called me. It may sound cruel to be thankful for my friend's misery, but the fact that I had eight children to care for (six of them under age 5) was a blessing to me as the next days and weeks went by, waiting and praying and hoping that Lenny would wake up and be okay.

"When that wonderful day came, and Lenny regained consciousness, Emmie called me and put Lenny on the phone. I remember how weak his voice was, but he knew me, and told me he was eating ice cream. I knew nothing, absolutely nothing, about head trauma injury. I truly thought that soon he would be himself, the Lenny we had for those 17 years, because clearly God had answered our prayers – we had our Lenny back."

"What I wanted for Lenny John was all wonderful … the best that I could dream of. Now I know that he was destined for so much more than my finest imaginings could have ever conjured," she says.

Over the years prior to Lenny's injury, Hannah had developed a drinking problem that only she and Emmie and a few others knew about. She had been praying to God for help. Praying for Lenny felt different than praying for herself. She began to realize that God had answered her prayers, that he'd given her Lenny back, but that she had to take care of herself in return. And, so, she went to her first AA meeting. She had heard about the 12 steps before but they had never registered. Now they did.

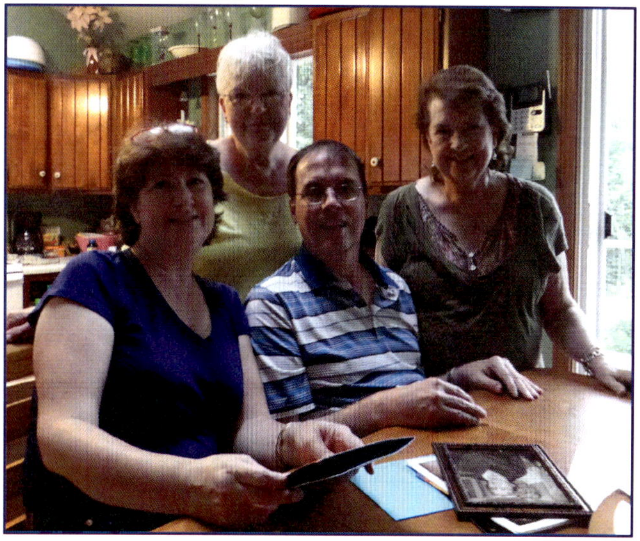

Cousins and sisters: Jessica Franzoni, her mother Hannah Bondioli, Lenny and Emmie.

When she told Emmie what she was facing, Emmie wanted to fly out to help her; that's what she had done when they were little and what she had done all her life: taken charge when there was a problem. But Hannah had to do this on her own, trusting in the help of her God. She checked in for residential treatment and went through a program that has helped her remain sober all these years.

That "enabling" of Emmie's began when they were young children living in Ticonderoga, NY. Once, when Hannah was about six, she brought a butter- and sugar-coated slice of bread out to the paddock for her Shetland pony, Nemo, who promptly inhaled it along with Hannah's finger. Hannah knew that if she tried to pull out her finger, she might lose all the skin and so she started screaming for help.

"I can see my mother in her housedress and apron and Emmie running behind her, yelling 'Get out of my way.' She ran up to us and popped that horse in the nose; he opened his mouth and my hand was free. She said to me, 'You've got two hands. Why didn't you just pop him yourself?'" Hannah recalls. "She was always not just doing what needed to be done but teaching, teaching, teaching at the same time."

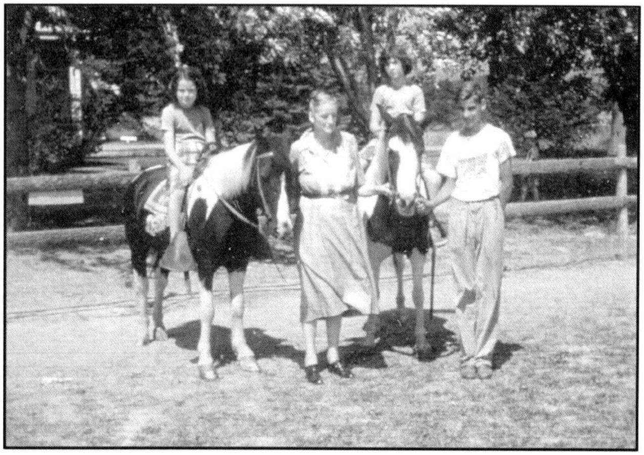

Hannah on her Shetland pony, Nemo, Dorothy Ormsbee, Emmie on her Welsh pony, Queenie, and a cousin, John Webster.

The girls' elderly father died when they were 11 and 9 and their mother, Dorothy Ormsbee, decided to move to Chittenden simply because she had fallen in love with the town after going to a flower show there. She bought a house they all loved although they had to use an outhouse. Taking care of the house and working was too much for her, however, and much of the responsibility for raising Hannah while earning a bit of money fell to Emmie. Throughout the teenage years, says Hannah, who concedes to having had a bit of a wild streak, Emmie was the one who protected her from herself.

"The many obstacles along the way, for Em, were simply challenges to surmount," says Hannah, who now lives far away in Wisconsin, but likes to visit Vermont each summer. One year, shortly after Emmie and Lenny started Lenny Burke's Farm, she too began working there. It all happened because her husband had told her it was time she got a job. As a mother of six, she hadn't worked much outside the house. "I said, 'Good luck Joe. I can bake, sew and make a great loaf of bread.'" Well, of course, these were all skills that were needed at the farm.

Leaving her husband for the summer "was a very independent thing for me to do. I thought the sky was going to fall. People worried that I would get a divorce. It really helps to know that I have people that love me so much that they were willing to give me a job."

Lenny, the first child born to the sisters, has continued to inspire Hannah over the years. She says, "Lenny's cheerful attitude is a gift to everyone lucky enough to know him. During his recent time of conquering cancer and enduring chemo, when we'd talk on the phone, it was always 'I'm fine Aunt Hannah, don't you worry about me. I'm doing great.'

"Then when I was home a year ago, hoping to be able to help out with his recovery from reconstructive surgery after the cancer operation, blood clots hit his lungs, and instead of the projected surgery, he was in excruciating pain. Yet we had to urge him to tell us, so the meds could get on top of the pain instead of chasing it. And he was joking with the doctors and nurses and aides. Strange circumstances to look back on as a good time, but Lenny and I had such a fun time in that hospital, together for a whole week."

These are the blessings of a life, says Hannah, the widening circles of family and strength, making life better through positive action and sharing the lessons learned from tragedy with others.

Traumatic Brain Injuries (TBI) Signs and Symptoms

Traumatic Brain Injuries (TBI), especially mild TBIs or concussions, can sometimes go unrecognized. A TBI is caused by mechanical forces that immediately and temporarily disrupt the normal functioning of the brain (e.g., car crashes, falls, abuse, sports). The mechanical trauma that causes a TBI may be either a direct blow to the head, face, and neck or an indirect blow elsewhere on the body that transmits an "impulsive" force to the head. A TBI also results in immediate neuro-chemical changes within the nerve cells of the brain.

People who sustain TBI's or concussions may experience symptoms over several days or weeks before these symptoms resolve. Ongoing symptoms after an TBI or concussion may indicate a more serious TBI.

After any TBI, it is always best to see a physician and/or be evaluated in an emergency department, especially if there are any signs and symptoms.

Common signs and symptoms after a TBI tend to cluster in two major groups: cognitive and behavioral symptoms, and physical-sensory symptoms.

Cognitive and Behavioral Symptoms may include the following:

Confusion, feeling in a "fog"

Getting mixed up with time and place

Having difficulty with attention and concentration

Inability to do more than one thing at a time

Having trouble with memory and forgets things

Having slurred or irregular speech

Having trouble understanding or organizing words or thoughts

Becoming impulsive, acting without thinking

Becoming restless or irritable

Becoming upset easily

Becoming sad or depressed

Becoming anxious or nervous

Physical or Sensory symptoms may include:

Headache, dizziness, light-headedness

Vomiting or nausea

Sensitivity to light, noise and activity

Numbness, tingling

Fatigue, tiring easily, drowsiness, problems falling or staying asleep

Blurry vision

Ringing in ears

Balance problems

Seizures

Any of these signs or symptoms after a TBI are RED FLAGS and should not be ignored. Seek help from a medical professional as soon as possible.

recently. But, he told his mother, he wanted to do more.

Lenny often accompanied his mother on her field trips to schools, homes and other places where she helped develop learning plans and otherwise provided support to people who had sustained head injuries and to their families. For many patients and caregivers, seeing Lenny mobile and happy was proof positive. Many knew his story and drew hope from his recovery, albeit limited. As for Lenny, he loved Emmie's idea that they create a "home" for people like him, people who could learn from and support one another, people whom his mother, Rev and her small army could help to become more independent. He began talking with her about making that dream of hers come true.

But Emmie knew she needed to finish something she had always wanted to do first – to return to school and earn a college degree. The idea of four years in school seemed daunting, however, until Emmie learned about Johnson State College's program of giving credit for life experience. Well, she sure had that. Gathering the troops, she elicited letters attesting to her knowledge and proficiency in a wide range of academic subjects from music education to science. Kathleen Ledo, the nurse from Rutland Hospital who'd told Emmie to stay calm when Lenny had first opened his eyes, had at the same time observed Emmie ask sophisticated and complex questions about anatomy, physiology, hypothermia and brain pressure. In her letter to Johnson State College, she praised Emmie's ability not only to learn about the body and its responses but also to do so during a most difficult time. Dr. Upton, the naysayer, wrote a letter in which he talked about speaking alongside Emmie at the first National Head Injury Foundation meeting held at the Rutland Hospital in 1982. He said he considered her an equal in knowledge and understanding of the complex issues inherent in treatment of such individuals. He particularly wanted the college officials to understand that Emmie's decision to return to school had as its ultimate goal not personal accomplishment but to ensure "that others will not have to go through the rather fragmented care that her son did." Of course, Emmie didn't tell him that, yes, getting a college degree *was* about personal accomplishment. Emmie was about to step even farther from the comfortable role of wife, housekeeper and mother and she wanted to be taken seriously in doing so.

In all, she got close to a dozen letters attesting to her capabilities and knowledge about the brain and head injury, treatment and rehabilitation, and letters that praised her organizational and planning skills. Based on these and Emmie's report on her own activities, Johnson State College awarded her 107 college-level credits, an exceptionally high amount given for life experience. Of course, in most cases, these were experiences she'd rather have done without and there were thirty units remaining before she could collect her degree. Which she did, of course, graduating from Johnson State College with a bachelor's degree in special education in 1984, one year before her son Kevin received his degree.

"Lenny took full credit for my degree," Emmie says, laughing as she explains that "He sat at the table with me and I would tell him what project I was working on. I would ask him to help me. It was a lot of writing about my life experiences. As we worked together, I could see how much he did remember and what he still struggled with. I also got to see his strengths. He *should* take some credit. I wouldn't have been in that situation without him."

HIS Independence Project, Inc.

Help for Head Injured/Stroke Patients & Their Families

Corporate Sponsor: **Killington Ltd.** Corporate Sponsor: **Mintzer Brothers, Inc.**

THE VERMONT CHAPTER OF THE NATIONAL HEAD INJURY FOUNDATION (NHIF)

2nd ANNUAL 24 HOUR MARATHON

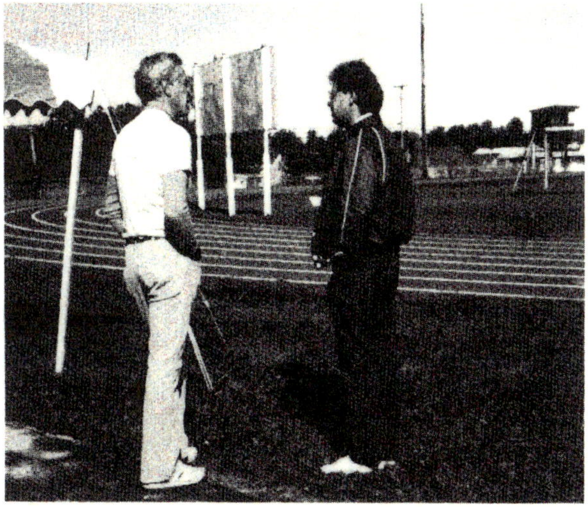

Bernie Buteau (Chairman of Development) and Ron Savage (Co-Founder of HIS) chat at the beginning of the marathon.

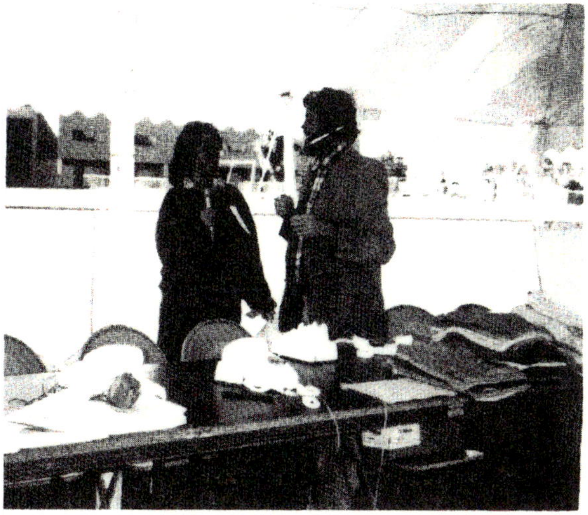

Jeff Phelps (Board of Directors) and Emmie Burke (Executive Director) discuss some highlights of the 24 hours on WHWB. The tent sheltering them was donated through the generosity of Taylor Rental Center.

On October 12 & 13 of 1985, Dr. Bernie Buteau ran 95.5 miles in 24 hours to help raise over $6,000 for HIS Independence Project (for head injury/stroke) in a one man 24 hour marathon. Our 2nd annual 24 hour marathon was held on Saturday, September 27th to Sunday, September 28th from noon to noon at the Rutland Vocational Technical School on Woodstock Avenue in Rutland.

TED WILLIAMS BECOMES HONORARY BOARD MEMBER OF HIS
LENDS HIS SUPPORT AND INTEREST TO PROJECT

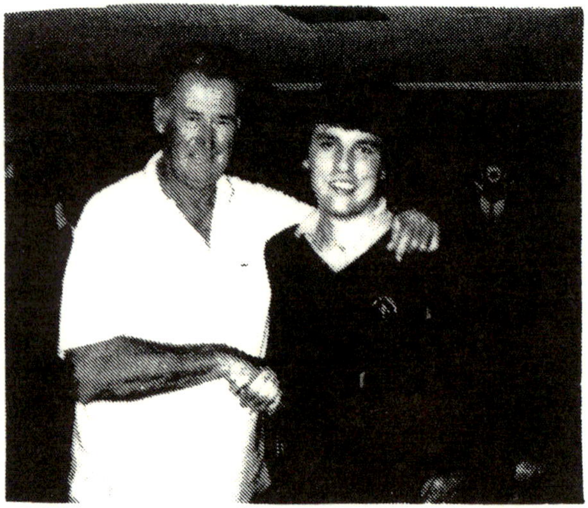

Ted Williams, former Boston Red Sox leftfielder and member of the Baseball Hall of Fame, became acquainted with head injury and its effects when he visited Lenny Burke last fall. Lenny, who calls Williams the greatest hitter in the history of baseball, suffered a head injury seven years ago while playing basketball for MSJ.

Pledge Your Support

TO: HIS INDEPENDENCE PROJECT, INC.
P.O. Box 1837
Rutland, Vermont 05701

Telephone: 802-773-2649

And so, in October 1987, armed with her degree and the conviction that a home-based therapeutic environment would be best for people with traumatic brain injuries, Emmie bought an old farmhouse on Route 7 in Wallingford that had a big barn where she envisioned craft classes and animals for the clients to tend to, each according to his or her abilities and inclinations. Actually, the mortgage on the farm was initially in her husband and son's names. Emmie had applied for a grant from the federal Office of Special Education Rehabilitation Services to purchase it, but was turned down, although she did receive a very nice letter suggesting she apply again once the farm was up and running.

It soon became apparent, however, that her husband was not going to join her and Lenny on the farm as had been discussed. By now, Emmie was getting used to operating on her own, so she and Lenny just moved there together and began setting up the big farmhouse for clients. Eventually, she and Len made an agreement that he would keep their house in Mendon and she would have the farm. After that, Len and Emmie remained friends but considered themselves separated for several years; they divorced in 1990. Of course, after Len's name was off the mortgage, the bank (she declines to name which one) demanded a cosigner and a male at that if she were to have the mortgage in her own name. She had signed the house in Mendon over to her husband in trade and, thus, couldn't use it as collateral. Fortunately, a friend came to her aide as a co-signer, someone she's also disinclined to name.

So much for women's liberation ... but Emmie's time would come.

As he has gotten older, Kevin, who now manages Lenny Burke's Farm and its satellite buildings and programs, has come to understand the depth of his mother's undertaking. Here was the woman with the beautiful pianist's hands "leaving the house on the hill and the in-ground pool" to live in a drafty farmhouse that she would heat with wood that she would transport in her suburban station wagon and chop into kindling herself. Of course, she'd had farm training as a child in Chittenden but that had been a long, long time ago.

In an article announcing the purchase and founding of what she called Lenny Burke's Farm, Emmie was quoted as saying, "We trust our instincts. We know exactly what we want to do here. Why wait to do it?"

Less than two months later, on Jan. 1, 1988, Emmie and Lenny – then her only employee – got their first client, a young man named Erik Searles. Searles had been recommended by the Independence Center. According to his high school friend, Penny Paquin, Searles had lived a "charmed life, a man out of a Ralph Lauren ad" until his accident in 1977. His grandfather had been a mayor of Newport, located along Vermont's northernmost border, and Searles himself had been a star athlete at North Country Union High School, much like Lenny Burke. Searles' father, a pilot and a jeweler, had died in a commercial plane crash on Moose Mountain in Etna, New Hampshire, on his way home to his son's football game. His brother, Robert Searles, says Erik always wanted to fly himself, but he began drinking early and had three DUIs before his accident, making him an unlikely candidate for flight school.

Searles was in the intensive care unit in what Paquin describes as a "wakened state of coma" for a long time, then spent the next 10 years in various treatment centers, including the out-of-state Greenery Rehabilitation Center. For a long time, his brother says, Searles lost the ability to speak and, on several occasions, was fed through feeding tubes because of aspiration issues. Eventually, due to the high cost of the out-of-state facility, he was placed in a nursing home in northern Vermont, which is where Emmie Burke found him.

Robert Searles was optimistic that his brother, who had gotten off to such a difficult beginning, might have another chance at Lenny Burke's Farm as its first client.

And, says, Emmie, "Erik was delighted, too. He was out of nursing homes he'd been in for 10 years. He was quick to tell us that he was a daredevil and it didn't take us long to learn he was telling the truth. He was honest about his background. He was quite rugged despite his disability. He could easily swear and get his temper up but he had a great sense of humor and under his brusque nature had a sweet heart and we loved him. We discovered that he really wanted to live a normal life again even though he resisted a lot of our attempts to help him get independent. That's what happens to people when they are in a situation where they can't do much for themselves for a long period of time. They start to believe they can't do anything. But we used his own desire to be independent as the tool to get him there," Emmie recalls.

Another small chapter in the story had also come full circle. About the time that Emmie was moving to the farm, Rev had decided that he wanted to do more for mankind and had accepted the call to go to Haiti to work with the sick and impoverished residents there. This meant giving up his various ministries and it also meant that Ellen, a person who loved her home and gardens, which she kept impeccably

Vanessa Doggett

They're singing Vanessa Doggett's song, "Brown-eyed Girl," a Van Morrison classic, at the weekly group meeting at Lenny Burke's Farm. The 38-year-old woman is wearing her new favorite outfit, pink top and pink leopard print Capri pants, and clearly enjoying the music, even though she can't join in vocally.

Doggett cannot sing or talk for that matter. But she can hear quite well and signals her joy with a thumbs-up sign, then points to her own clear brown eyes as the group sings, "Yes, you, my brown-eyed girl."

Doggett's mother Marie describes her as a "wild child, the first female wrestler at Burlington High School. She loved colorful clothing, loved to dance and sing and party, and play the violin." That is, until she nearly died in a horrible car accident on North Street Extension on Dec. 7, 1995.

Her girlfriend, Vicky Roy, was at the wheel. The two had been drinking at Alley-Cats, a restaurant and bar in Burlington, even though Doggett was underage. At the time, the 19-year-old Doggett worked three jobs – at Daffodil for her clothes, at a local printers for rent, and at an exotic dance club for spending money. The details of the traffic accident remain elusive as Roy died instantly. What is known is that Roy and Doggett appeared to either be racing against or trying to escape from two men driving in another car. Police said the speedometer on Roy's car stopped at 113 mph when it crashed into a tree and split in half. Doggett was not found right away, as she was thrown 150 feet from the vehicle. Medics revived her three times before she was transported to the hospital. Her brain was injured in five places.

Doggett has limited movement in her limbs and has difficulty swallowing, requiring a feeding tube. Despite these obstacles, she communicates using a

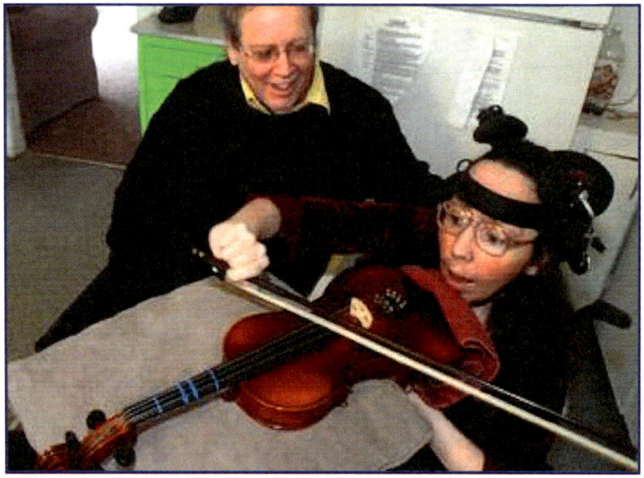

DynaVox communications device. Over the years, with the help of Gary Miller-Wade, a life skills aide who leads the weekly group sessions, she has also tried her hand at playing her old favorite instrument, the violin, along with a lap steel guitar, an autoharp and many percussion instruments, all in an attempt to provide her with outlets for her musical creativity.

According to her mother, Doggett was given less than 48 hours to live when doctors finally evaluated her. "They called her a living vegetable but I didn't believe them. I knew she was in there. I said, 'If you understand me, I want you to blink, once for yes, twice for no.'" Her daughter blinked once. She then asked her to give a thumbs-up sign for yes and a clenched fist for no. One day she put a pen in her daughter's hand and Doggett started to write.

Her mother could only do so much, however. Enter Emmie Burke, who heard about Doggett through her social worker at Burlington Health and Rehabilitation, the third treatment facility Doggett had been placed. The social worker, Erin Weaver, had noticed Doggett cry when she heard that a favorite singer had died. She thought the young woman was too bright to live the rest of her life in what was essentially a nursing home and worked hard with Emmie and Kevin to have her transferred to Lenny Burke's Farm, where she lives at Emma's Place.

At the same time, Kathy Chandler, a local woman who had been working with people with disabilities for years, was hoping to get a job at Lenny Burke's Farm. Its philosophy fit well with hers and, as it turned out, her expertise in working with clients who required tube feeding and exercise that incorporated a full range of motion was exactly what was needed if Doggett was to move to the farm. The two came together in May 2000.

Doggett had a "dinosaur" of a communication machine when she arrived. The one she has now stores important information and her writing projects. Says Chandler, "She's a pro. If we have someone new to a DynaVox, we sit them next to her and she does the job of showing others how to use it." Doggett is currently writing her autobiography on the machine. Born Feb. 17, 1976, she's calling it Bicentennial Baby.

Chandler says her mobility has improved since coming to the farm. Her left arm is contracted but the right one has improved enough that Doggett can create craft items with beads and yarn.

She loves going to the lake nearby, using the swim cart that Chandler's husband created. The story of how this swim cart came to be illustrates the way things happen at Lenny Burke's Farm. Staff wanted an easier method of transporting clients to Elfin Lake, but pushing them across the shoreline and into the water was difficult using wheelchairs. Swim chairs for people with disabilities cost about $30,000. One day, when his wife was working overnight, Mark Chandler stopped by to play cards with the clients, and heard about the problem. He started studying photos of new ones and took an old bathing chair of Doggett's, adapted it with pressure-treated wood that wouldn't rot, outfitted it with balloon tires and voila. And it all comes apart for easy transport. Now, on summer days, many clients get to go "swimming" in Elfin Lake, equipped also, of course, with life vests.

These days at group, when the other clients summarize how they are feeling and rate their mental and physical health on a scale of 1 to 10, Doggett is likely to write a rather eloquent and sometimes bawdy offering that her machine recites for her in a confident female voice.

One day last spring when the weather had finally turned sunny and warm after an exceptionally long and cold winter, Doggett's message went something like this, "The weather has become a good, wholesome environment. Opinions are like assholes; everyone has one. But I've been working out and keeping my body looking good. The weather and my body have given me a moral boost. I am a 20 today."

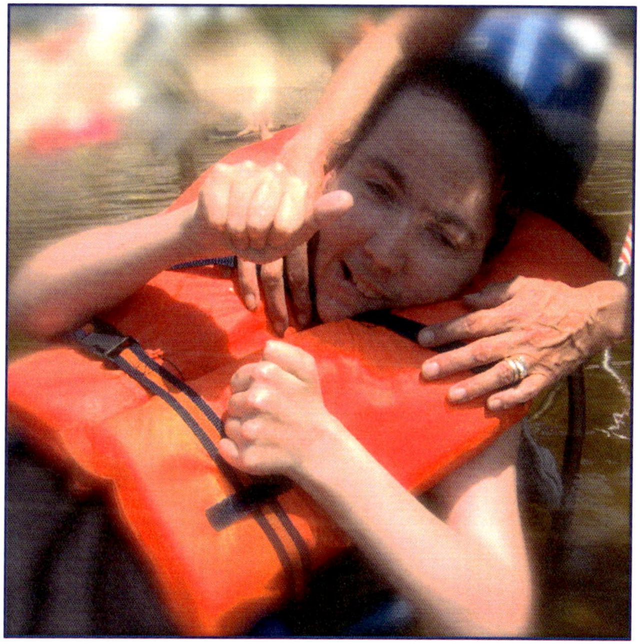

Vanessa Doggett "swimming" in Wallingford's Elfin Lake.

clean, would accompany him to the island country. As might have been predicted, it was too much for the couple, no longer youngsters and unused to the very harsh conditions under which they were living in Haiti, and they returned home to Vermont with needs of their own. Soon enough, they were both working at Lenny Burke's Farm and, as Rev put it at the time, he'd found "his new mission right in my own backyard."

Searles had tremendous tremors and a host of physical problems that kept him confined to a wheelchair, yet he hated that he had missed out on a lot of life. Once, Emmie stopped at a car wash while she and he were out grocery shopping. The carwash scared him half to death; he'd never been in one before. "He hated that I'd seen him scared. He was proud," she says. Searles and Rev got along beautifully. In those days, Rev, who was quite tall, still maintained his athletic grace. (COPD slowed him down before his death in an automobile accident in 2010.) One day, when Rev was trying to get Searles to help peel some potatoes, Searles made a bet that Rev couldn't put his foot in the sink without holding onto something for purchase, that he couldn't just stick it in from a standing position. Rev did it and Searles had to peel the potatoes.

Robert Searles remembers visiting the farm and commenting to Rev, "'Jeez, he's different,' and Rev said, 'Yep, he's gotten sober.' It was true. Even when he was in a nursing home, he'd found ways of getting alcohol but now he was sober because he wanted to be."

Says Emmie: "Erik was a challenge but it was a joy to watch him gain new skills every day. We didn't care how long it took him to do something; we just encouraged him to try something new every day. We did well together and I was learning from him while he was learning from me, but we were in desperate financial situation. We needed another client if we were going to make ends meet. And then this family came to see us."

The family Emmie is referring to is that of Yvette and Ezra Bashaw who had been praying for a treatment center or home in Vermont for their son, Dick Bashaw. Bashaw was 33 years old in 1984 when he was bicycling home from a bike race and a car passed him just one-quarter mile from the road to his home in St. Albans. Perhaps the driver who aimed to turn down that road didn't calculate how fast Bashaw, then the second fastest bicycle racer in Vermont, was peddling. He could easily do 35 mph. The driver and he collided at that intersection; Bashaw was thrown 15 or 20 feet. His bike helmet fell apart upon contact with the road and the right side of his skull was crushed. He still bears the indent in his head.

Bashaw eventually ended up at the Head Injury Center at Lewis Bay in Hyannis, Mass., quite a challenge in terms of regular visitations from his family. His mother heard about Lenny Burke's Farm from the national brain-injury group, came for a visit and immediately fell in love with the farmhouse, especially the homey kitchen that Emmie had decorated with old plates and cute curtains.

Initially, it appeared that Searles and Bashaw were opposites – Searles' head injury was on the left side while Bashaw's was on the right, and they had opposite personalities. Searles liked rock 'n' roll and jazz music while Bashaw, who'd been brought up in a very religious family, sang hymns and Christian songs. Searles was loud and had a temper; Bashaw was quiet and didn't like uproar. But what they both enjoyed were the things that made Lenny Burke's Farm different from so many other centers and institutions where people with disabilities or injuries are housed or treated, the family atmosphere, the home-cooked meals, and activities that both taught necessary skills while also being fun or at least tolerable.

"I told Emmie right away, right off when I met her that I like to eat," Bashaw says. "And Emmie, she is one good cook."

Like Searles, Bashaw also took to Rev. As a result of his injury Bashaw had painful hammertoes and other limitations to his mobility. His toes were bent downward, making walking very painful. Also, like Searles and so many people who sustain serious head injuries, he struggled with short-term memory loss. But he had a strong desire to recoup his athletic abilities and to regain his cognitive skills and so he took on whatever speech, memory or physical exercises Emmie or Rev offered. That in turn motivated Searles, who didn't like to be left behind. And Lenny, who played endless card games with the two of them and sang both the rock 'n' roll songs and the Christian hymns, served as motivation for both men, almost joyously taking part in whatever arts and crafts lessons or balance exercises were being offered on any given day. Lenny was a natural in this regard, relishing in sharing memory strategies that he had learned for himself much as he had enjoyed teaching Kevin the Pledge of Allegiance. He had many small jobs as well, which helped with his self-confidence, from emptying the wastebasket to setting the table. Indeed, he got up every morning prepared, as he put it, "to go to work."

All this, in turn, helped Lenny to talk better, to remember more, to control his spontaneity, and to laugh at himself when he couldn't do something. Within a year of being at the farm, the University Health Center clinic where he had been having routine evaluations since the year of his injuries noticed a marked change in his physical health, his communication skills and his emotional demeanor. Among the improvements discussed in the clinic's report that year were his ability to note his own mistakes and correct them coupled with an improved ability to stay on task and carry on a more complicated conversation without repeating himself. As Lenny recently expressed it, reflecting back on those first years at the farm, "I was helping our clients realize who they were and how much they could do without having to pass a big test. The only tests they had were with themselves. And that in turn was helping me. I had a purpose."

Emmie immediately got Bashaw into treatment with a podiatrist and followed through with recommended therapies and exercises. Not to be outdone, Rev started sharing silly foot jokes with Bashaw and the two quickly developed a repertoire. Dinner would be punctuated with conversations that went something like this: "What does an elephant do when he hurts a toe?" "I don't know. What?" "He calls a toe truck!" Or, "What makes a podiatrist happy?" "I give up." "Hearing the pilot say, you are now approaching 20,000 feet."

Emmie knew that Searles was a little jealous of Lenny but one day he surprised her with this confession: "He said, 'I wanted to tell you why I hated you. I thought you brought Lenny to the nursing home to see me because you wanted me to see what I could have been like if *my* mother had lived.'" His mother had died a few years after his injury, according to his brother who noted their closeness.

Emmie responded this way: "'No, Erik, I brought Lenny here because I didn't want to leave him at home.' And then he said, 'I know that now.' And I said, 'Erik, I know you are getting better when I see you do something nice for someone.' The next day, he told me, 'I did something nice. I gave your son a candy bar.'

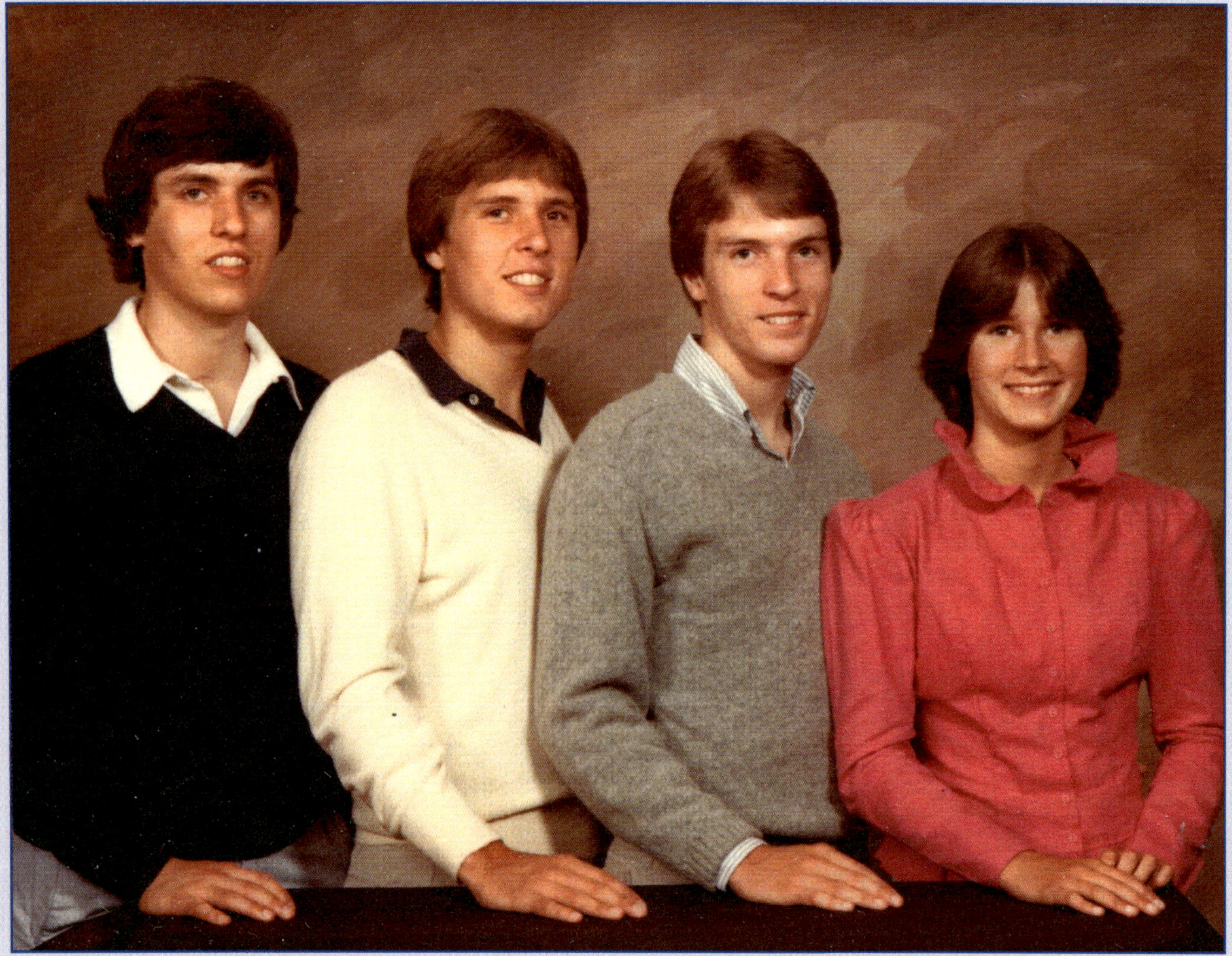

Lenny, Kevin, Michael and Kathy Burke.

The Bend In the Road Becomes the New Road

By Kevin Burke

When out of state friends visit me here in Vermont, I am always sure to take them to the Chittenden Reservoir. It is arguably one of the most beautiful places in Vermont. One hundred acres of pristine, swimmable water, surrounded by spectacular mountain vistas, including a great view of Pico Ski Area to the east. On its western slope sits an inn, where you can have lunch or dinner, cross-country ski, snowshoe, sled down the hill, or even take a horse and sleigh ride. Summer means swims at the beach, kayak, paddleboard, or even taking a pontoon boat around the reservoir. Growing up in Chittenden we did all of these things and more.

I tell my visiting friends, as we enjoy our meal, or kayak, or swim, the same story (it's my story and I am sticking to it!), that while I loved growing up the way I did, at the time I never saw the incredible mountain views. Whether it was the naiveté of a child, the intense focus on activity, or just thinking that every place was that beautiful, I never noticed the view. Didn't everyone have that natural beauty surrounding them while growing up? These days, I can't drive from my home to my office without ogling the surroundings. It's not just the foliage season that we are known for, or even just the snow-capped peaks of ski season. Our area of Vermont is incredible all of the time, even in the off seasons.

That's a little bit like what I experience in trying to write a memory of my brother Lenny. As his (our) journey continues, it's easy to see clearly his wonder. As his 19-month-younger brother, he was just always there. His face was peering into my crib when I was an infant. He was there when I took my first steps, encouraging me along. He taught me how to run, how to swing a bat, ride a bike, (and before this, much to my mother's chagrin again, how to pee down the old heat registers in our bedroom, so that we wouldn't be caught not sleeping during nap time!). He was an ever guiding presence. My wife has blown up a favorite black and white picture of us from that time in our cowboy outfits: hats, holsters, boots and all. We spent happy hours and days playing in our Chittenden home. Fishing, swimming, playing baseball and basketball, sliding in the winter, riding bikes (his was always blue, mine as the younger brother, red) When he was going to go to kindergarten, my 3-year-old self heard my parents, aunts, uncles and grandparents talking about it excitedly (our home was filled with family and friends). I thought this was great, and since I always tried to emulate everything that he did, I assumed that when the old yellow school bus showed up in our driveway at summer's end, I would be on it with Lenny.

Shocked and saddened when I learned that fateful morning that he was to get on the bus without me, I burst into tears. I dressed myself in my favorite cowboy boots, without socks, my navy blue overalls with my pajama top, and tried to stomp onto the bus. I was not to be dissuaded. My parents unsuccessfully tried to calm me down and get me from trying to make a break for the bus. Nothing was working until Lenny himself, aged 5, told me not to worry, that when he came home each day he would teach me and tell me everything he did and learned that day. I acquiesced. Then I held him to it.

Today, having been blessed with a beautiful 5-year-old granddaughter who has just started kindergarten, I am so conscious of how exhausting it must all be. Ready with a hug, a snack, a beverage, and ideas for fun the minute I pick her up on the days that I do, she is ready to relax a bit.

I am quite sure now that Lenny was too. Cookies maybe. Anyone that knows him knows that you do not come between him and his cookies. For him certainly some outdoor play with definitely a ball (football, basketball, tennis ball, baseball, he did and does love them all!) involved. A nap even. It was not to be. His determined (stubborn?) 3-year-old brother was waiting for him daily, holding him to his promise of teaching me the day's events.

Teach me he did. Under his constant tutelage I arrived at kindergarten well prepared when my time came. Teach me he still does.

Lenny's character, then, and now is impeccable. He made a promise, he kept it, even at 5.

It's really hard to write about memories of Lenny without bringing up his athletic ability, and for that matter his proficiency at almost anything he turned his hand to. He could climb the highest on the tree and jump off without getting hurt. He was an expert fisherman, both brook and still water. His aim and strength of his throw, honed from many hours of practicing baseball, was such that, amazingly, he stunned a 16-inch brook trout with just a rock. We pulled it out of the water, and brought it home to clean and fry. We had slingshots, and watched Daniel Boone on television. We always had dogs as pets, and in my case horses. Although incredibly allergic to horses, Lenny, not surprisingly, was a great rider. I would groom and saddle the horse; Lenny would jump on and go for a fast gallop on the quiet Chittenden roads. Upon his return, he would jump off quickly, getting out of his clothes and into the shower as quickly as possible to avoid an allergic reaction, while I dealt with the horse. We were a team. When we were very little we had rabbits, and would look forward to Sundays all week long, when, after our bath, provided we had been good, we could bring the bunnies inside with us while we watched Walt Disney.

I suppose, like not seeing the mountains, that I thought everyone had a big brother like mine. I don't think I ever truly took him for granted; he was always just there.

Lenny continued to try his best to teach me and set an example through our elementary school years. I am not claiming I always followed said example. Our growing up was, of course, not without the occasional spat and sibling rivalry. I remember one wresting match in particular, where somehow my head ended up going through the slatted door of our closet. Oddly, we did not share a room for very long while growing up. I couldn't wait to have my own when my father, a building contractor, expanded our home. Somehow I ended up with my own, and he shared his with our younger brother, Michael, who needed a big brother like I did. That's the kind of brother he was, and is.

When I was in 6th grade or so, we were studying the frontier age in history. We studied the politics of the era, read pioneer testimonials, and as a final project, for which we had weeks to prepare, were to construct a replica of a pioneer settlement. Our natural surroundings lent themselves to making this project easy, and fulfilling. The soil, rocks and sand, twigs, brush, and even some implements that could be found in our barn would have made this a fun project to work on. Had I worked on it.

The night before it was due, just as bedtime came, I finally told my parents about the assignment. They were not happy. Lenny, always earlier to bed than I (a trait that has served him well) was already almost asleep.

Hearing my distress, he immediately offered to help, offering his Lincoln Logs as a solution. Maybe not as good as the natural materials on our property, but pretty good thinking by my 8th grade brother. My father was so mad that he didn't want Lenny to help, saying "Why should he be up late for your mistake?" Lenny didn't see it that way. He loved me, and wanted to help me avoid a pitfall. He leaned down out of his bed, and worked on the Lincoln Log village with one hand, until my parents relented and let him get out of bed and help. That's the type of brother he was, and is.

Following in his footsteps to high school, it was a lot of fun being his younger brother. He had made his mark with sports, especially basketball and golf right away. Because I enjoyed other things, namely skiing, a lifelong pursuit of mine, while he played basketball, it was easy not to be jealous of him. He made this easy by being the way he was, and I celebrated his success. This is not to say that I was not experiencing the usual teen angst, rebellion, and making the normal inroads at breaking away from my family of origin at the time. But always, I was happy for my brother.

Very early in my high school career, January of my sophomore year, the moment came when he almost was not there.

Sitting in the bleachers on January 23, 1979, I was enjoying the game with some ski team friends. That it was Lenny's senior year, a winning season, and him the highest scorer in the Southern Vermont League all contributed to making the games very well attended and exciting, with many eyes on him.

The moment he was aggressively fouled, and hit the backboard, then the old parquet floor of the gym, an enormous collective sigh came over the entire gym. Although none of us could possibly know just how much at that moment, anyone present was aware that something horrible had just happened, make no mistake.

I think that because of the type of student, athlete and person that Lenny was, and also the fact that this was not a reckless act on his part with drugs and alcohol involved, the community support started immediately. The support was meaningful, incredible, far-reaching, and continues to this day with my mother and our efforts to help others with brain injury.

Because the worst, death at age 17, did not happen, the journey has never seemed to be as bad for those around Lenny as one might expect. He was spared, and we were relieved and happy to have him in our midst. So much good has come from this tragedy. However, I would never be so arrogant or presumptuous to speak for Lenny. It is he who has fought the battle, he whose life was forever altered that January night.

In large part because of my mother's strength, and her willingness and capability to not only care for Lenny, but work toward sharing with others, I was able to go off into the wild blue yonder for a bit, and pursue my own goals with college and travel. When I returned to Vermont in 1989, Lenny Burke's Farm was up and running. Rev and my mother invited me to stop by Wallingford and visit while I was on the way to a job interview in Manchester.

I have been here ever since, and have been a co-director since 2001, after many years of career tutelage spent with my mother and Rev. Just this summer I became the director so my mother could partially retire. I have tried to never take for granted this gift of being with my brother and family, while doing work that I love. It has been an incredible way to spend my days for the last 24 years. As the saying goes, "How we spend our days, is, of course, how we spend our lives." In this instance, I know that I have chosen well.

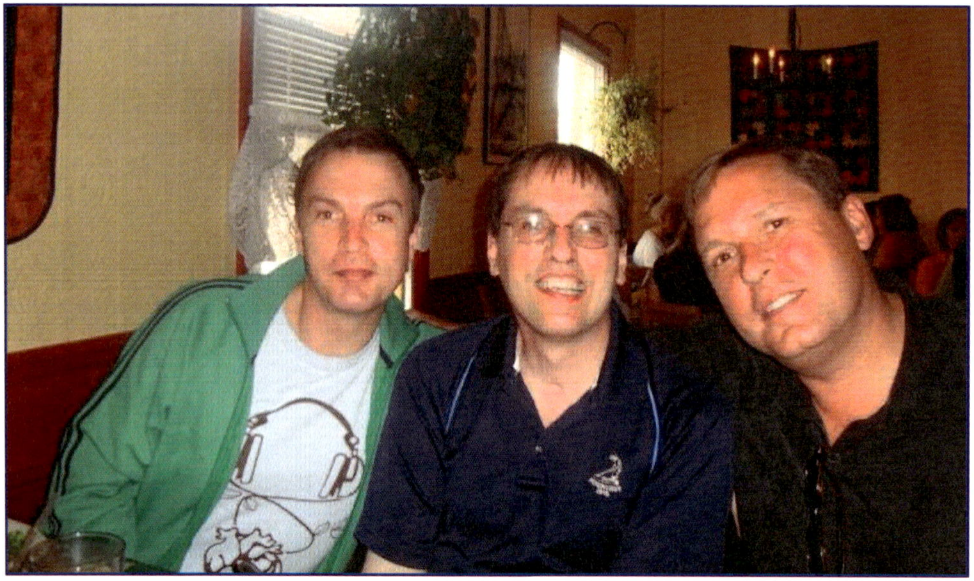

Michael, Lenny and Kevin Burke.

Lenny remains, as described in Vermont Magazine, "a sunny and optimistic presence at the Farm." Always the older brother and good example, as well as a coach, he brings his skills to all who come to the farm community.

In 2012 lightning struck again. I had just been at an elementary school reunion where everyone was asking about Lenny. I was so proud to tell old classmates and friends about Lenny's present life. Six days later, our dear, caring staff rushed him to the hospital with severe abdominal pain.

Another vigil. Two days later my mother, my dear aunts, and my wife and I were standing in a surgical waiting room at the same hospital awaiting news.

It was cancer.

How could we not flash back 34 years?

The reaction of everyone who receives this news is nearly identical. Oh no! Why him? I admit, over a year later I still have these thoughts.

Not Lenny. His immediate response? "I don't think, why me? I think, why not me? And just work on getting better"

Amazing.

The next year was filled with more pain for him, pain that I would rather feel myself if I could take it away from him. After many years of absence, my father became a huge support during Lenny's surgery and chemotherapy. They spent a great deal of time together from August until March, with my father visiting daily and often taking Lenny to his chemo appointments. My father entered hospice care one day before Lenny's final chemo. He died March 18, 2013, peaceful in the knowledge that Lenny was fighting the good fight, and would overcome yet another battle.

And Lenny has. He's now cancer-free and very much alive.

The "Old" and the "New" Lenny

By Michael Burke

Lenny was an ideal older brother. We shared a room growing up and although I was four years younger than him he never made me feel like the little kid. He was incredibly supportive of all of my interests – my artistic endeavors, my menagerie of animals that we kept in the room, my passion for the sciences.

I received constant encouragement from him. He had a quick wit and a dry sense of humor and I have no doubt it's where I got mine. Lenny took great pleasure in me being able to "hold my own" with his friends, joining in with a sarcastic or cutting response at the appropriate moment. He was smart, funny, and athletically gifted. He provided a road map for me of the type of person I could aspire to be. His passions inspired my passions.

I was thirteen years old when Lenny was injured. I wasn't at the game and when Gail Austin picked me up that night from a friend's house and told me he had been hurt, I thought he had broken his leg. Gail didn't say it and it wouldn't have mattered because I'd never heard of a head injury before. None of us had.

The next morning when that terrible, remarkable, photo of the moment that Lenny was pushed was in the newspaper and I read the article, I knew it must be serious, but there was something in my thirteen-year-old mind that allowed me to hold on to hope, to expect that he would be OK. Perhaps it was a lack of life experience.

The next month and a half was a whirlwind of crises, grief, and heightened emotion. People were at our house all day every day, dropping off food and making sure we were all right. There was a constant vigil of our school friends at the house and we had massive sleepovers on the living room floor. It was a tremendous outpouring of community support.

After forty-six days, when Lenny emerged from his coma and started speaking to us, it was nothing short of a miracle and my thirteen-year-old self was sure that this meant he would now fully recover despite the fact that Lenny at this stage, because of the extent of his injuries, was much like a two-year-old. He had no inhibition, he talked almost constantly, he was unable to walk, and his eyes were unfocused. But this, I was certain, was only temporary. When you break your leg, they fix your leg and after a time you return to normal. Surely this type of healing would hold for a head injury.

We brought Lenny home and soon he was off to Burlington for rehab. I trusted that he would get better but progress was slow - nearly imperceptible. Then when mom found the famous Rancho Los Amigos rehab center in Downey, CA, I was sure that this would be the answer. These were the people who would "fix" Lenny.

The plan was for him to stay six weeks. With my mom gone for so long the house quickly fell into disarray.

At the end of the six weeks, Mom called to say the therapists wanted him to stay six more. I thought it was a good sign. They just needed more time to fix him, to make him exactly as he was before. My 11-year-old sister Kathleen, in an effort to fill mom's role, burned grilled cheese sandwiches for dinner every night. It was a difficult time but we were focused on the outcome and Lenny's recovery.

So three months later, Dad and I flew out to pick him up. I couldn't wait to see Lenny, now fully recovered. I was going to get my brother back. When I walked into the hotel room, my heart sank. Lenny was there, but he was talking "inappropriately" and his physical deficits were still evident. I couldn't see any change at all from three months prior. Suddenly, the full impact of the extent of his injury and his life after hit me. There would be no fix. Lenny would never be the same again. Ever.

Anyone who has been touched by traumatic brain injury knows that the person is the same and not the same. You have to learn to mourn the loss of the person who is still in the room with you. It's a strange, long process.

Once you reach acceptance though, the world opens up again. And you find a new normal. Our "New Lenny" is just as remarkable as his old self. He is our sage, our family spiritual advisor, the life force of our family. I have never met anyone more positive than him. It's humbling. He is incredibly courageous and very easy to love. He is still my role model and a role model to countless others.

Many TBI survivors lose subtlety but Lenny never did. Thankfully, he never lost his incredible sense of humor. That's how we got through it. Lenny taught us how to deal with the aftermath of his injury and his humor helped us all to keep it light.

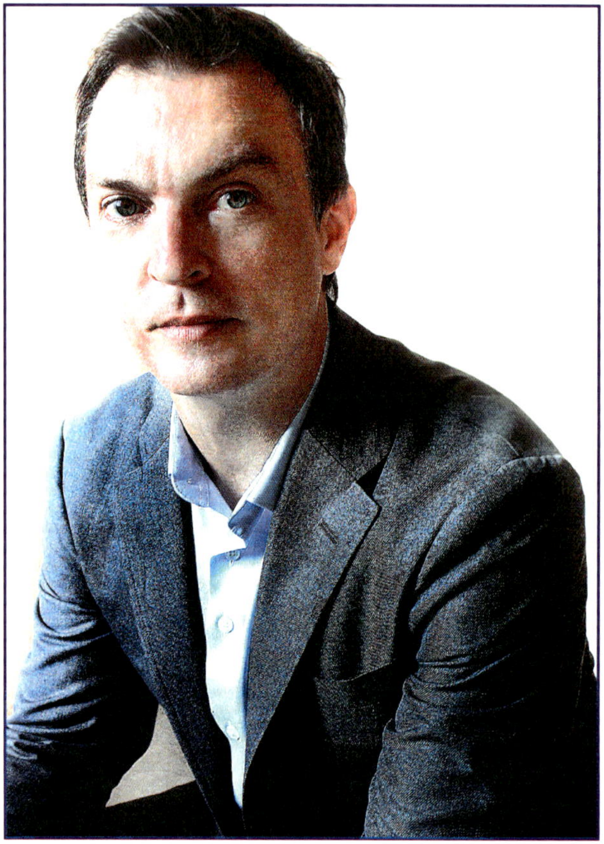

Michael Burke.

My mom reminds me of a time in the early days when Lenny was upstairs taking a nap. Mom and I were downstairs and we were looking at Lenny's beautiful senior picture hanging on the wall. I said to my mom "If Lenny woke up and was the old Lenny – the one in the photo – I would miss the new Lenny."

That's even more true now.

> "Lenny is incredibly courageous and very easy to love. He is still my role model and a role model to countless others."
>
> *–Michael Burke*

Life Lessons

By Kathleen Kourebanas

My childhood wasn't typical. Some say it may have been cut short. I have never felt like I missed out on anything. I feel I experienced life just as I should have. My mom is my hero, of course. I couldn't have asked for a better role model. And Lenny is the sweetest angel you will ever meet. You have to know him to hear his genuine soul in his soft voice. He fills my cup every time I see him.

"Kath, have I told you what a great sister you are? Do you know how proud I am of you and what a great mom you are?" is just a sampling of the beautiful accolades I get to hear every time we see each other. Lenny is a gem of a man, he is rare and he is so precious. I absolutely adore him. I still drive him a little crazy and bug him like a sister should. He gives it right back. Anything that I may have missed out on in my childhood is given back tenfold in the beautiful moments I have shared with my family.

It's hard to describe the affect that Len's head injury had on me. I think to say it simply, it gave me great tools that I would need in life. Maybe at age 10, I didn't realize it but now at 46, I am grateful for all the difficult times we have had as a family. I do get compared to my mom a lot. We both married men who ended up not being our life partners. We both have beautiful children. We both put our kids' needs before our own. And we both make fantastic lemonade out of the proverbial lemons life has given us. I like to think of Len and my Mom as my best friends now. Of course, they are family too but I can barely go a day without talking to my mom and sending my love to Len.

There were a few pivotal moments that helped mold me early on. I remember taking Len grocery shopping soon after I got my license. Some kids in the store parking lot started mocking him and how he almost lost balance getting out of the car. I confronted them, gave them a piece of my mind and then proudly held my brother's hand as we walked into the store. I imagine I'm not the only sibling in the world who has had that experience. It's empowering but it's also scary. It was scary as I felt I needed to protect my brother. But with age comes wisdom and I soon realized that ignorant bullies don't matter. Lenny taught me how to stick up for people, to say the least. He gave me a view on life that I would never have had without him. It has come in handy as I raise my two children.

My beautiful boy, Tommy, loves his Uncle Len and YiaYia Emma. Tommy has never seen Lenny as having a TBI. He doesn't notice that he walks with a gait; he doesn't notice that he has short term memory loss. He does notice his love of sports and how much he loves his family. Lenny is a wonderful role model. He often tells Tommy how lucky he is to have me as a mom. Tom always responds, "I know Uncle Len." They share a love of basketball, the Celtics, of course. And they love Sunday football games. It warms my heart to see them watch a game on the couch together. Tommy, like myself, has had lots of exposure to people with disabilities. He isn't fazed. One of my proudest mom moments was watching Tom buy a homemade piece of artwork from one of our clients in a wheelchair who used a Dynavox to speak. As a young boy, Tom looked at him, spoke and waited patiently for his response. It was beautiful. Lenny helped give him that confidence, patience and acceptance and that beautiful skill of seeing the ability and not the disability.

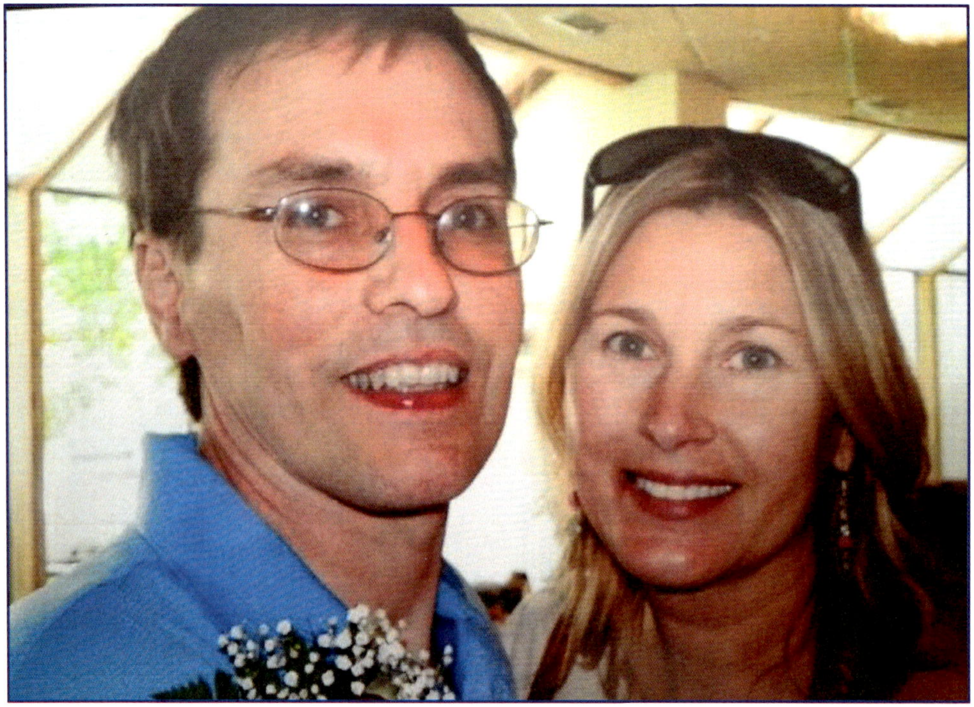

Lenny Burke and Kathy Kourebanas.

My daughter Martha has struggled her whole life with social anxiety and challenging behaviors due to autism. My mom has been my rock through it all. I don't know where I would be without my Mom's guidance and support all these years. Martha needs constant care. TBI and autism are quite different, as people are. But Martha will need support and supervision throughout her life, as well. So as I follow in the footsteps of my hero, I've decided to open a home for Martha. It won't be a residential care home but simply a shared supported home for Martha and a roommate. Martha is nearing 15 and won't live there for a few years. So in those years, I'm starting a nonprofit organization on the land surrounding her future home. Martha Emma's House (tribute to both of her loving YiaYias) will share its three-acre property with the local autistic community. On the property will be a barn, greenhouse, chicken coop, and walking loop. My plan is to open up group and individual activities, vegetable gardening, animal care, egg gathering, exercise, and weekly social events for Martha's peers. And who knows, these activities could turn into jobs one day. It is so needed. Just like Lenny Burke's Farm was years ago.

"Lenny is a gem of a man, he is rare and he is so precious. I absolutely adore him."

—Kathy Kourebanas

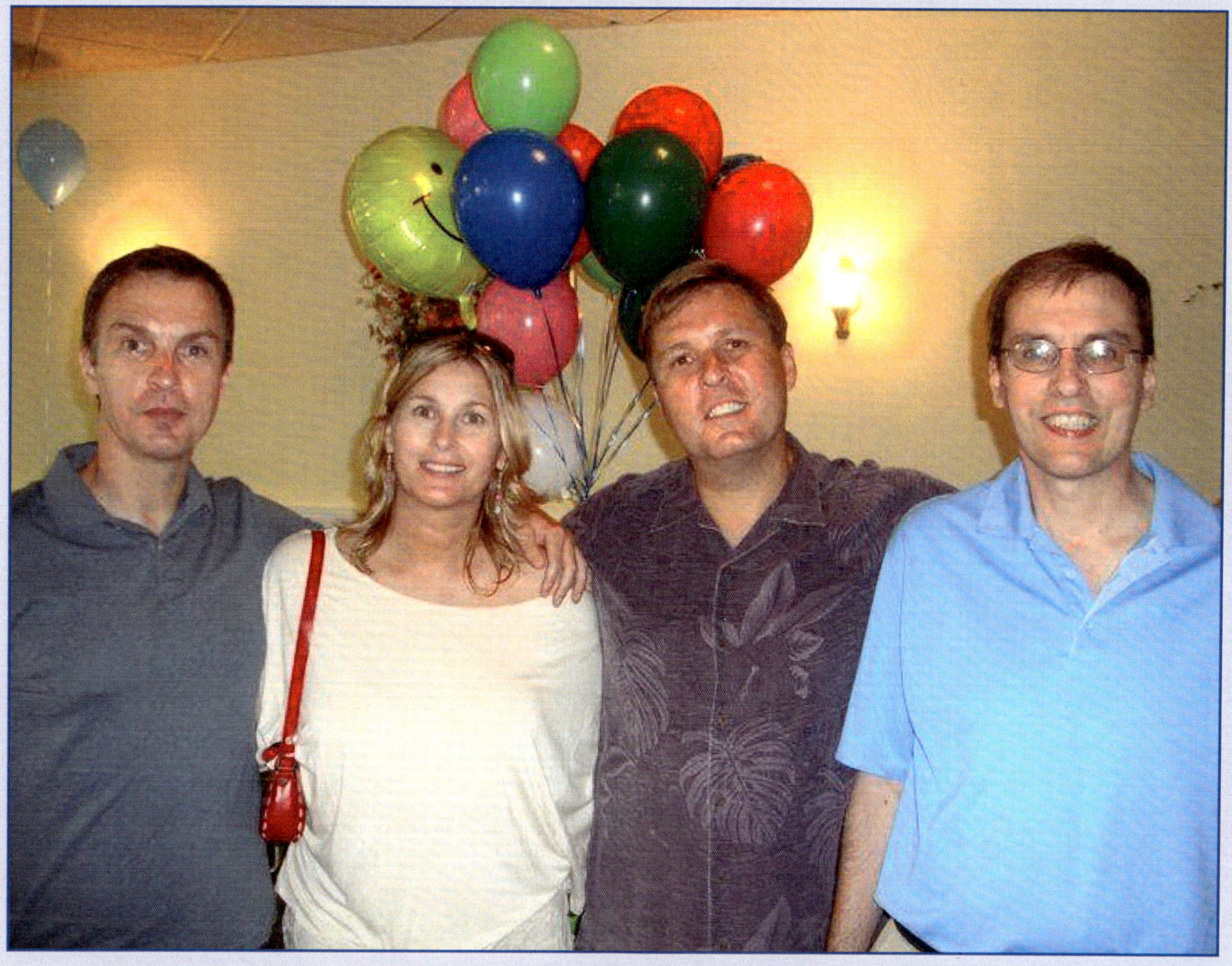

Michael Burke, Kathy Kourebanas, Kevin and Lenny Burke at Lenny's 50th birthday party.

"It just melts your heart," says Emmie, recalling how those early clients showed her how lucky she and Lenny had been to be surrounded by a supportive community. It's also easy to see how such a deep admission on Searles' part helped Emmie to understand the despair experienced by many people whose lives have been limited by a head injury. She had no idea that Searles had any ill feelings toward her. And perhaps it was easier for him to express himself that way, rather than admit his jealousy of Lenny, who had progressed so much further than he. She also more fully realized the benefits Lenny had reaped from being surrounded nearly continuously by people who propped him up and kept him moving forward. Unlike Searles, he'd not experienced that deep despair. But people like Searles and Bashaw, who had been housed in places with few stimulants and little hope of progress, would need a lot of help seeing the future in the best possible light. In that, Rev was especially useful. Just as Lenny had been able to talk to Rev as a young boy first questioning life's complexities, Rev had a way of meeting each client where he or she was. You have to love a person who drives around in a car with a bumper sticker that reads, "I wish I could be the person my dog thinks I am!"

About this time, Dr. Johanna Ruess, a physiatrist from the Medical Center of Vermont, called about a third client, a woman named Brenda Shores, who had a poor memory, the result of a car accident when she was 19 that had left her in a coma and in the hospital for several months. Dr. Ruess thought she was a perfect candidate for Lenny Burke's Farm, seeing in her the potential to improve and live independently. Shores would be Emmie's first female client, but before she could accept a third client, she needed to get licensed as a level-4 rehabilitation center. Dr. Ruess was so impressed with what Emmie was doing and convinced that there were more people who could benefit from a home-based therapeutic center such as hers that she helped Emmie get the required licenses.

Shores, too, was more than relieved to finally get out of an institution. Emmie was pleased at how well she got along with everyone. Shores represented another success: Her rehabilitation progressed to the point that she was able to get a job at the nearby Cumberland Farms store and eventually graduated from the farm, married and had two children.

From then to now, there has never been a shortage of clients, many referred to the farm by state agencies, schools, hospitals and people working in nursing homes and rehabilitation centers. Then as now, the staff follows the philosophy Emmie applied to Lenny: provide a safe and wholesome environment that as closely as possible resembles a home with good, home-cooked meals eaten together; involve clients in their own care; lead each to increased independence through repetition and reinforcement, building skills all the while; and involve the clients in games and activities that stimulate their minds while providing reasons for them to keep trying harder, whether the impetus is winning a game or watching a garden grow. All this is supplemented with carefully monitored and individually designed use of resources available in the wider community – medical care, physical, vocational and occupational rehabilitation, and counseling services. Contact with family members is encouraged and many clients go home for vacations, holidays or special occasions. But for those for whom that isn't possible, birthdays, holidays and anniversaries are a reason to celebrate together.

Kathy was involved with the farm from the beginning, working as a life-skills aide and later as a one-on-one support person for various clients, including Eric Searles. Her employment at the farm was almost accidental. It happened because Emmie had a meeting she absolutely had to attend to and couldn't fathom how to take Lenny, Bashaw and Searles with her. Kathy volunteered to stay with them. When Emmie objected, Kathy said, "You do it, don't you?" Perhaps a bit of a wisecrack but when Kathy retorted in a most self-confident voice, "Then I can do it, too," Emmie realized that Kathy had been studying how to help people with traumatic brain injuries from the moment of Lenny's injury. And so Emmie hired her daughter. Kathy was involved with the farm in various capacities when she wasn't at college from then until 1997, when she married and moved to Essex to care for her two children, Tommy, now 16, and Martha, 15.

Meanwhile, Kevin had graduated with a major in sociology and a minor in business from the University of Vermont, where he interned in Washington, D.C. for the late U.S. Sen. James M. Jeffords, then a congressman, and worked as head of interviews for UVM's admissions office. He considers his mother to be very wise, understanding that her children had had to accept grown-up responsibilities quite young. She supported Kevin's efforts to "pursue my own dreams" in his early 20s.

Kevin spent those years waiting tables and bartending in Chatham or on the Jersey shore, earning his college tuition money. After college, the big sky/big ski country drew him west. Winters were spent at Copper Mountain Ski Area near Vail and summers at the shore. But one day in the fall of 1989, his mother and Rev asked him to stop and visit the farm on his way from the family home in Mendon to a job interview at EQX radio in nearby Manchester, Vermont. Kevin had decided to spend a little time around his family and the job offer at the radio station had been enticing. Maybe his mother and Rev had something else in mind, however, because Kevin never made it to that job interview after he saw what they were up to at the farm and they asked him to consider helping with assessments of new clients.

"I just saw it, and then I got it," he says simply. He started working 20 hours a week, applying his organizational skills to the business of running the farm. He's been there ever since and became co-director in 2001. This past August, as Emmie stepped down to partial retirement, Kevin became the farm's director.

"I had no intention of working here, it was Mom's thing," he recalls. "I was proud, but not fully aware" of what the farm was all about. Looking back, "my college major, degree, internships, etc., all fit (with what was needed at the farm), but I never did it with that in mind. Mom is so gracious about saying how we helped her get started. Not me. I think it's important that it was her. I was skiing and at the beach. It all is her legacy."

As Kevin puts it, "Because of her, services in Vermont lead the nation. Other programs, many of which we helped get started and share a positive relationship with today, exist because of her. Emmie's dream was not just to have Lenny Burke's Farm, but to have a place for every person affected by brain injury in Vermont to go to … How many people has she inspired, women in particular? It's hard to tell but I know it's substantial."

One can say, however, that it was Michael Burke who actually made the place a farm. His college career at the University of Vermont had been interrupted in the early 1990s by a rare case of rheumatic arthritis caused by an undiagnosed strep throat and he had been recuperating at home. When he was better, he too spent some time traveling and experiencing life but when his travels wound back to Vermont, he found himself also drawn to the farm. In not too much time, Michael too was working there, helping with clients while attending Castleton State College. By now, Emmie had purchased a duplex where she and Lenny lived with some of the clients and was renting other properties in which she moved clients as they became more independent. Each of these clients in turn would be assigned an aide who worked directly with the client on tasks such as preparing and shopping for food, going to appointments and corresponding with families and guardians. Because the clients were close by, they could come by the farm for peer sessions, group therapy and other support services, as needed, and as most of them could not drive, they had someone to accompany them to doctors' appointments and rehabilitation programs.

Since the main property was technically a *farm*, Michael decided he wanted to raise animals, something he'd always loved. Indeed, he was the kid who always had pets – guinea pigs, rats and ferrets, canaries and snakes.

"Growing up in the country, you're supposed to show your tough side. But I always had this incredible empathy for animals," Michael recalls of his youth. A famous story involves one of his ferrets. Rev was visiting one day, wearing his signature dress pants with a sharp pleat up the center of each pant leg. A ferret ran right up his pants. "It was an act to behold, him releasing the ferret from his pants," laughs Emmie.

Dicky Duck, a Muscovy, had come with the farm and then there was the chicken that Emmie kept hearing in the barn but could not find until the day Kathy stayed to take care of the clients. When Emmie returned from her meeting, Kathy told her that she kept hearing a chicken clucking and it was driving her crazy. Together, they climbed up to the third floor of the barn, following the sounds, and there they found a chicken that had apparently been surviving on its own for some weeks. Of course, they adopted it and fed it well – until a few months later when they asked the farmer across the road if he happened to be missing one and, seeing a chicken filled out quite nice and plump, he said, "Why, yes, I did and it was the nicest one I owned. That's it right there."

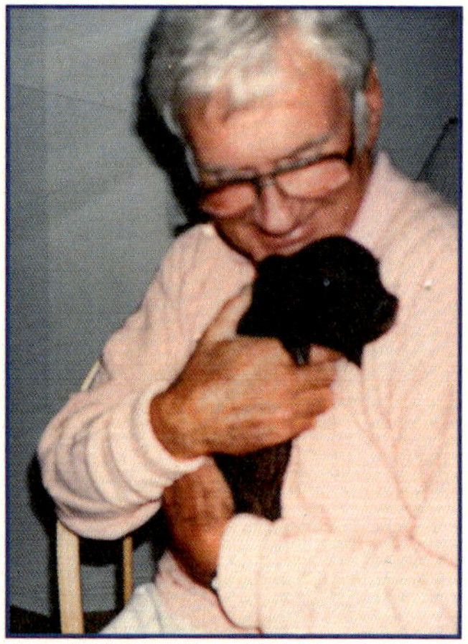

Sid Davis, a former LBF co-director, with one of Michael's baby pigs.

Some of Michael's animals weren't exactly your quintessential Vermont-type critters – especially the pot-bellied pigs he decided to raise. Of course, they're cute and people raise them as pets but they do get big. One of the female clients so associated Michael with the pot-bellied pigs that she called him Pigman because she couldn't remember his name. Michael also had a regular pig that Kathy thought was "the cutest thing walking on high heels" until the day she came home from college and inquired about the pig. Appalled when Emmie said she was going to have to give the pig away, she was getting so big, Kathy went to see for herself. When she opened the barn door, a 300-pound porker lunged at her. Off the pig went to the neighbor across the street, with the promise that the family would not eat her. One day, Emmie got a call from him: "You are the proud grandmother of 13 piggies." This provided another lesson in rural reality as the farmer told Emmie that the mother pig only had 12 teats. "Once a piglet grabs onto the dinner plate, no other pig can have it," he told her. "But not to worry, the mother pig sat on the extra one and now everything is fine."

Fine until Emmie got a book about small farming and decided to raise some sheep, which came as adorable baby lambs. Fine, she thought. I love lamb, too; we can do this. Lenny went right down to see them and immediately named them Rambo and Lambo.

When Emmie said, "I can't kill and eat Rambo," Rev's wife Ellen, a woman who had a less sentimental view of farm animals than Emmie, replied, "I can and I can cook them for you, too." There were pigmy goats, too, named Emmie and Hannah, for Emmie and her kid sister, now all grown up and living in Michigan.

And horses. And dogs. And cats. Everyone's welcome, it seems, at Lenny Burke's Farm.

When Emmie and Lenny envisioned the farm, they knew their clients would have a wide range of capabilities, that some would need lifelong care and support and that others might eventually live on their own; still others would need a combination of independence and support, perhaps living in their own apartment but with the assistance of an aide who might help with setting up medications or taking them shopping and to doctors' appointments. In 1996, Lenny Burke's Farm became one of the first facilities to gain state approval under Vermont's innovative Supported Apartment Program, aimed at creating a real safety net for people with disabilities who wanted to live in the least restrictive environment possible.

Searles, Bashaw and Shores all achieved this level of autonomy, moving from the farm, to assisted apartments and then to their own places. Searles was the first.

"Coffee helped Eric get independent," Emmie recalls a bit wistfully. "He had tremors and huge physical problems. But he got around fairly well in his wheelchair and could certainly learn to make his own coffee. He knew it and he knew I knew it. But he would get everyone else, especially Rev, to make his coffee for him. Not Ellen. She'd say, 'Eric, you can make your own coffee if you want it so bad,' and she showed him how. She was right, of course. Eventually, he learned how to do it on his own and, suddenly, he discovered he could do a lot of things; microwave meals, take care of his hygiene, do laundry. Once he saw what he could do on his own, he loved it."

Searles progressed quickly, moving from the farm to a supervised apartment and then into his own apartment in Rutland in 1990. In this setting, he blossomed. But there could be problems, the result of frustration and confusion, which in turn were manifestations of his head injury. For example, Searles liked to do his own shopping but maneuvering around clogged aisles would try his patience or he might have a terrible temper tantrum if the store's layout had been drastically altered or an item was moved from what he considered its "proper spot."

Of course, the grocery staff would not know what to do with him or even why he was so upset, but they learned soon enough to call Emmie for help. She'd get on the phone with him and say something like, "I'm so sorry they have done this to you, Eric. I'll ask them to put everything back exactly the way you think it ought to be." Searles would get it, that he was being unreasonable, calm down and finish his shopping.

Despite his occasional temper tantrums, Searles had an active social life. He made new friends in Rutland; staff from the farm who had grown quite fond of him continued to visit him. All that came to an end on his 38th birthday, Aug. 22, 1991. Robert Searles had attended a pizza party for him the day before and given his brother some birthday money and a new pair of sneakers. The next night, he was home in his apartment on Burnham Avenue when two men broke in, cut his phone lines, stole his money and gifts and, when he resisted, strangled him with his own belt after knocking over his wheelchair. He was very strong and police said he'd put up quite a battle.

His family and the Burke family took his murder hard; it was inconceivable that Searles had done so well only to be killed in a vicious robbery for just a few dollars. It was especially hard on Kathy who had worked closely with him.

"We all knew what his schedule was all the time," Emmie recalls. "Kathy had made him seven whoopee pies for his birthday, one for every day of the week, and almost stopped to see how many he had eaten that night, but didn't for some reason, and has always felt guilty that she didn't stop." Of course, Emmie is quick to point out that Kathy might have been there when the men broke in and that she too could have been murdered.

Fortunately, Bashaw's return to independent living went smoothly. He benefitted from strong family support, especially from a brother who converted a house for him so he could be close to his family. After going from the farm to a supervised apartment, he eventually moved back to St. Albans and got a job as custodian at Bellows Free Academy in St. Albans from which he will retire in June 2015.

Once a month, though, he travels to Wallingford to attend monthly socials at the farm. "I owe my independence to Emmie and Lenny Burke's Farm," he says.

Then as now, most of the farm's residents participate in some kind of life skills training, along with craft activities that range from art projects to woodworking. In the early years, they sold their work at a craft store located in the barn above the farmhouse at Lenny Burke's Farm. But one cold night in January 1996, a fire destroyed the iconic-looking barn that had drawn Emmie and Lenny to this property. Several of the animals died in the blaze, despite efforts by former Constable Nelson Tift to save them; the craft store, too, was destroyed.

But, as happens so often, especially with anything associated with the Burkes, this loss turned into

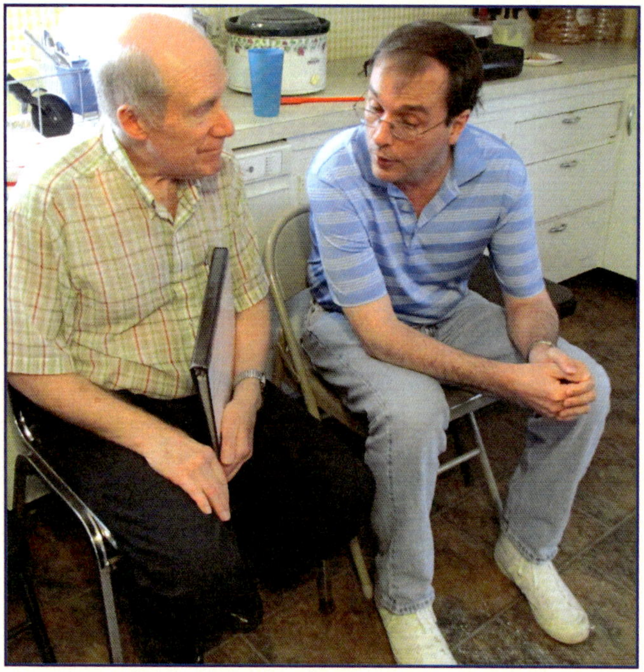

Case manager Hugh Barclay talks with Lenny Burke at a recent group meeting.

a new opportunity. Not long after the fire, in May 1996, staff member Butch Towsley, noting the loss of the barn coupled with the farm's growing clientele, suggested that Emmie purchase his mother's former home in "downtown" Wallingford.

Towsley's mother Emma had died the previous October; her property, now known as Emma's Place, included a large house, two barns and a third outbuilding. (This time, Emmie did not need a co-signer to purchase it; she'd proven her reliability to the banking establishment!) Together, the new buildings provided the needed room for arts and crafts, an office, and more residential space. (The barn at Lenny Burke's Farm was rebuilt but not into its initial three-story size. While there are still horses, goats, chickens and bunnies at the farm, the focus on animal husbandry has not expanded since Michael graduated from Castleton in 1994 and moved to New York, where he earned an MFA in film production from NYU.)

Most important, the purchase of Emma's place provided a second big home with lots of bedrooms for clients. Its oversize kitchen and generous living room allow for group exercise and Thursday group meetings. These days, Gary Miller-Wade, a talented guitarist whose work life has consistently revolved around two things – playing music and caring for people with disabilities – leads the weekly group gatherings that Rev initiated and ran until the week of his death. The highlight of "group" is an hour-long sing-along that features the clients belting out songs by the Grateful Dead, Golden Earring, Led Zeppelin, The Beatles and Pink Floyd or old favorites like "Danny Boy" and "King of the Road"

Sally Carleton, a talented singer in her own right, often joins in while Kathy Chandler, who manages Emma's place, takes over the guitar on "Stewball." Carleton is one of five former clients who now work at Lenny Burke's Farm.

As of summer 2014, Lenny Burke's Farm was serving 24 residents in its five staffed facilities; another 22 clients live in their own apartments with the help of the organization's case management services. Six clients, all male, live at the original building, a classic white farmhouse with red trim, just yards away from the barn that houses two miniature goats, a couple of bunnies, 14 chickens plus a rooster and two miniature horses.

Mike Joyce, a Tufts University graduate who manages the staff and clients living at the farmhouse, has worked in one or more capacities there for about 25 years. It was an incident that occurred at the farm when Joyce was applying for a job that convinced Emmie to hire him, even though he was fresh out of college with little experience working with people with disabilities. As it happened, she asked him if he would mind retrieving a kitten that wouldn't come down from the top branch of a tree. He did so with no hesitation and no second thoughts.

"I can use someone like him," she thought instantly. "He's strong, he's smart and he's not afraid of challenges – our kind of guy."

But Joyce, who was a longtime friend of Kathy's and a formidable football player at MSJ, wasn't quite sure he could work as a life-skills aide or plan menus. He joked that he could use some help with his own life skills or with organizing his daily activities, but Emmie knew he was a keeper. And when he said he could only make hamburgers, Emmie wrote on the menu for his night to cook, "Mike's extra special hamburgers," which expanded to include "Mike's extra special chicken," and, before long, Joyce could make just about anything special. Indeed, it was a good match as Joyce's no-drama personality and reliable, commonsense approach to the kind of daily challenges anyone working at the farm encounters has provided stability over the decades.

Erich "Buddy" McLellan
We All Have Hope for a Better Tomorrow

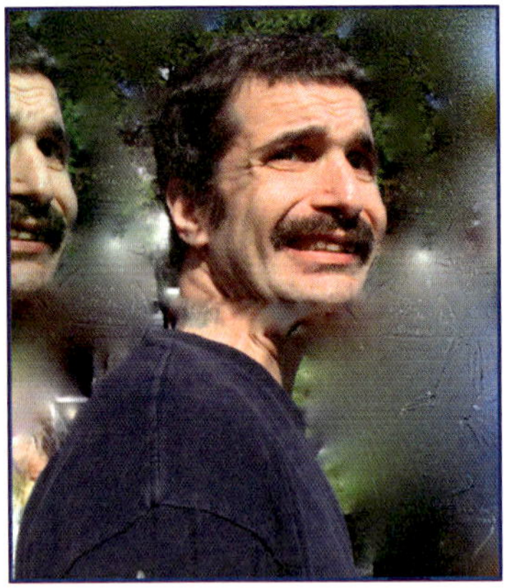

When Erich McLellan arrived at Lenny Burke's Farm, he displayed the kind of sheer terror visible here on his face. He rarely spoke and when he did, his words were barely audible. But, in the past year, he's begun to lose the fear that caused him to attempt suicide in 2009.

Below, he's reading the Lenny Burke's Farm's statement alongside John Shepard, a life-skills aide, and Jean McDuff, a client who lives independently in Rutland.

The words are: Recovery: Lenny Burke's Farm. There is no place like home. We are all family. A circle of friends. Everybody knows your name. Everyone in the circle respects each other. A circle of faith, love, harmony, hope and joy. Recovery: Nobody wins alone. Courage does not always roar. Sometimes it is

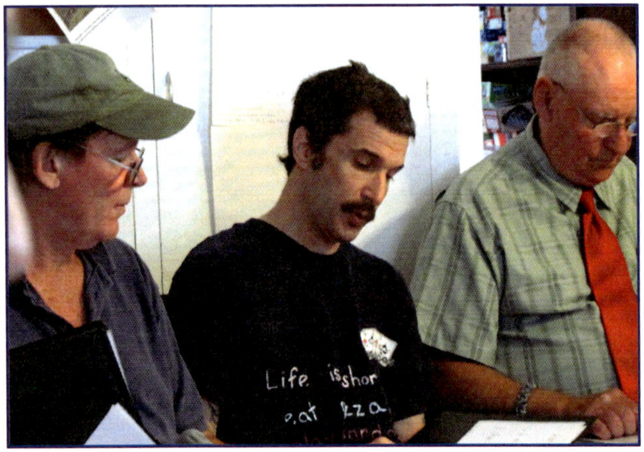

a quiet voice at the end of the day, saying, "I will try again tomorrow."

We all have hope for a better tomorrow.

Few know the depth of a parent's anguish as deeply as Judy Linn, who was told that her son, Erich McLellan, was not going to live after sustaining separate brain injuries three years apart. Indeed, Linn's daughter had just gone through the torture of identifying her brother's body after the second incident and was about to leave the hospital when she learned that a nurse had detected a heartbeat.

Says Linn of her son, who goes by the nickname Buddy, "He's one of the luckiest men in the world and that goes all the way to him somehow arriving at Lenny Burke's Farm. In a strange way, he's more of who he was meant to be now."

McLellan's teenage and young adult years growing up in Guilford, Vermont, were difficult, she says, explaining that "Buddy was a really sweet baby, but he was severely dyslexic and didn't fit in. He struggled with school and always wanted to be a tough man. He was a biker and got lots of tattoos but he just wasn't that way. We knew that but he was trying to compensate for his disabilities."

His first brain injury occurred in June 1976 when he 24 and driving drunk. He lost control of his car and somehow hit a parked dump truck going backwards about 80 mph. The accident occurred on a deserted stretch of Route 5 just across the Vermont border with Massachusetts. Fortunately, an EMT worker who was driving by saw the car or McLellan would have died from those injuries. His recovery appeared quite rapid but the next few years were a mess of relationships and some legal difficulties that suggest he'd had more serious brain damage than initially thought.

McLellan, who had two sons from two relationships, was sent briefly to jail where his mother believes he had a psychotic break. He came out worse than when he went in, used heroin, got involved in another relationship, had more charges brought against him and was sent to jail again.

"At that point his behavior was very erratic. He kept saying he wasn't going to go to jail again. Whatever happened that first time really terrified him. And so he hung himself" on Thanksgiving Day, 2009.

Brain cells without enough oxygen will begin to die after about four minutes. Says Linn, "We were told it was between nine and 12 minutes before he was found. We were away at the time and my daughter was the one who was called to identify the body. As she was leaving the hospital, he was being transported to Dartmouth by ambulance" because a heartbeat had been found.

"It was an awful situation," Linn recalls. "My husband and I were told there was no brainstem activity. We had to make a decision. Days passed. After two weeks, we decided to take him off the machines and wait for him to die. Nothing happened. We waited another two days. Nothing. We were staying at a friend's house in Brattleboro when a big snowstorm hit. We couldn't get to the hospital, called to see if he was still alive and they said he'd suddenly started talking. We said to just give him water until we got there. And when we got there, Buddy was back, the Buddy we always knew was there. A sweet Buddy but a terrified Buddy. Terrified of going back to jail.

"I think when they unplugged him, it was like when you unplug a computer that's just spinning around. They rebooted him," she says. However, since the brain needs a constant supply of oxygen to function properly, McLellan suffered from cerebral hypoxia, which left him with a host of neurological and cognitive problems. He can walk but speech is limited and he remains easily frightened.

He was released from the hospital to Crotched Mountain Rehabilitation Center in Greenfield, New Hampshire, where he stayed until 2010 when he transferred to Lenny Burke's Farm.

"Lenny Burke took my heart and did for my son what I would have done with him if I had the ability."

—Judy Linn

Kathy Chandler recalls his arrival in late November, wearing nothing but sweatpants and a tee shirt. She took him shopping almost immediately; his first smile came when he got to pick out a sports cap. "We said to him all the time what we continue to say to him now: 'You're okay, Buddy. You're safe. You're home.' He was heavily medicated when he arrived and we worked slowly to wean him from his medications so he's far less lethargic. He's grown stronger simply pushing the other residents' wheelchairs. He loves doing that, that and singing the song, 'Them Old Cotton Fields.' He comes alive with that song."

Which is something that continues to amaze his mother who arrived for a visit last summer as Thursday's group session was getting underway. To hear her son, who could not read as a child, read the Lenny Burke's Farm statement in a clear voice with no hesitation over pronunciation amazed her.

"Lenny Burke took my heart and did for my son what I would have done with him if I had the ability. Going to Elfin Lake with him on that recent visit, I realized Bud has that quiet Vermont life you'd want for him. He has a life. He's not withering in a convalescent home. He's with people who care for him. He's blessed beyond anything I could imagine for him. He's treated with respect. My son is one of the luckiest men on earth."

These days, Joyce especially enjoys working with clients when they first come to the center, charting and following their progress as those who have had few incentives to learn independent skills get drawn into the farm's philosophy – fellows like Rich Martineit, who arrived almost incapable of doing anything for himself after years in which he'd been heavily medicated and suffered several medical setbacks.

Martineit's parents, Richard and Barbara, had moved to Vermont in 1997, the year after their oldest son graduated from the University of Connecticut. A brilliant computer engineer, Martineit was working for Cincinnati Bell Corp. in April 2000 when he decided to fly to Vermont to surprise his mother for her birthday. He only had the weekend home and his brother wanted to introduce him to his friends from work so one evening they went out to a party, stayed late, had a few drinks, and on the way home, the brother lost control of the car.

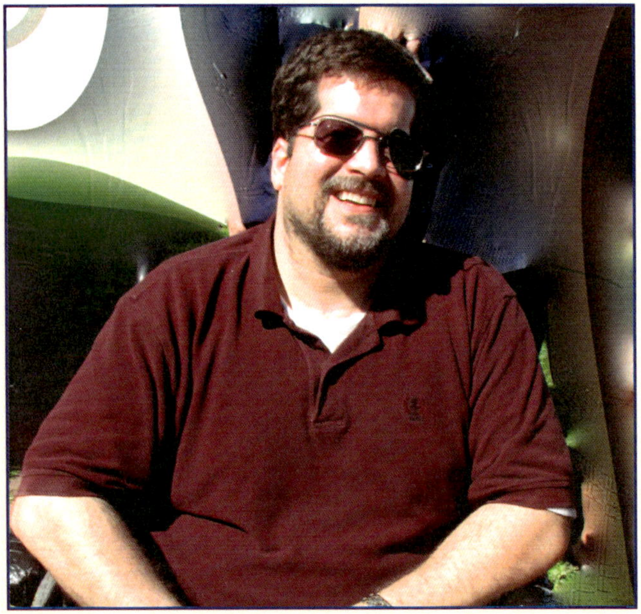

Rich Martineit.

Neither man was wearing a seatbelt but the brother's steering wheel had an airbag, which inflated while Martineit was thrown from the car.

It was the kind of situation that goes from bad to worse. Initially, Martineit was placed in a deeper coma, like Lenny, to facilitate healing; by then, doctors had learned to open the skull of brain-injured individuals to relieve pressure. He seemed to respond well when a piece of his skull was removed due to brain swelling. After a couple of months in the hospital, he went to Fanny Allen Health Care and eventually Crotched Mountain Rehabilitation Center in New Hampshire for further rehabilitation. Between 2000 and 2008, however, when he went to Lenny Burke's Farm, his speech and general abilities, which had improved over time, regressed when he developed hydrocephalies or swelling of the brain and his skull had to be closed back up so doctors could insert an artificial shunt to prevent the brain from swelling more.

Joyce, who has remained quite fit over the years, works with clients on basic life skills such as toilet use and eating, but also likes to bring those who can to exercise in the farm's workout room located in the barn. He knows that gaining control, if only partial, of one's mobility is good for one's outlook in life. Martineit is living proof. In the five years since he's been at the farm, he's gone from a fellow with his head hanging down and his eyes shut, incapable of doing anything on his own, to a bubbly man who plays on his computer, reads voraciously, and is gaining ground in walking by working out on a treadmill. Joyce likes to tell Martineit's story to new employees as an example of what can be accomplished through physical exercise, games, and patiently teaching clients how to do things for themselves.

Meals are especially important at the farm – almost as much for the staff as the clients as staff members spend long hours working with clients, some working overnight shifts and making the farm a second home. Linda Poro, who can basically open the refrigerator and with whatever she finds make something absolutely delicious, prepares most of the weekday meals at Emma's Place and sometimes cooks at the farm on weekends. When the guys there were going on one day about Thanksgiving dinners from their past, she went out and bought the ingredients, including a fresh turkey, cooked it up and served it to them on a Sunday afternoon, even though it was in the middle of the summer. Even she conceded it was the best turkey she ever ate.

Judy Gamez, who works at Emma's Place on weekends, likes to spoil the clients with homemade bread, brownies and chocolate cream pie along with traditional comfort food like shepherd's pie. And Denise Taylor-Clark, who began working at the farm almost from day-one and manages the building they call "The Duplex," located a couple of blocks from Emma's Place, designs her menu around what the residents, David Coffman, John Heir, Bob Savin and Mark Chaplin, love to eat, balancing healthy meals with an occasional treat.

Chaplin has been living at one of the farm's facilities since 1991 after he nearly died in the early 1980s when as a teen he smashed his car, traveling at speeds greater than 100 mph, into another vehicle. He had been drinking and was institutionalized in hospitals and rehabilitation centers for years before coming to the farm.

Because of his head injury, Chaplin had a temper and was difficult to manage; he'd occasionally threaten to run away even though he was primarily confined to a wheelchair. The staff devised a reward system to control his behavior, realizing that his injury had left him with problems with self control and impulsiveness. Back then, Rev was known to say, "I've got to find the Christ in Mark Chaplin." Emmie had a different tack. She'd warn, "I'm going to go get my camera so I can videotape you." That would calm him down; Chaplin had enough awareness to know he didn't want a record of his bad behavior. As with some of the clients, it was trial and error to discover techniques to keep Chaplin calm and happy; aging has helped as well, along with keeping to a daily routine with as little opportunity for anxiety as possible. In summer, he's happiest just sitting out by the creek watching the river flow past. And that bad boy who once gave Rev such a hard time now loves to help decorate a tree at Christmas and make sugar cookies with Taylor-Clark.

Hier is another client who needs special assistance because of disabilities from a TBI, a job that life-skills aide Michael Watson is adept at. Some times, it's not just helping with medications or meals; Watson takes Hier to visit his mother's grave when he asks.

But when there's a client like Savin, 72, who was hit by a car while working as a trash collector but has remained physically strong and active, Emmie's glad she has someone like Butch Towsley on staff. He not only takes O'Connor hunting and fishing and provides wood for him to chop and carve, but he gives Savin little jobs to do at either the farm or at his place in Tinmouth, tinkering with cars or working on the dock, all of which give Savin a little spending money. And when the clients go to Towsley's house for a day on Tinmouth Pond, Savin's usually the one who asks first to go tubing behind Towsley's boat. Savin, who has lived at the farm for 18 years, says "I like to work and keep busy. Butch knows what I can do and what I can't, and he's patient, which is what I need most."

Says Towsley, who retired from General Electric after 27 years in 1992, "I wasn't ready to retire and so

I started at the farm in '95. Over time, I've realized it is true that we can't give the clients all they want with their lives, the exact life they had before their injury and sometimes you do wish you could do more, undo what happened. But what you can do is make their daily life as enjoyable as possible. That's what I try to remember every day."

Since the farm's beginning, an estimated 300 residents have successfully taken part in its residential and therapeutic programs and moved to other settings. Many are employed, married or in a relationship; many drive and most live independently while others live in supervised facilities closer to their families. In all, the farm employs roughly 30 individuals, several of whom recovered from their own traumatic brain injuries through the farm's programs. These include Sally Carleton, Jim Fleshman, John Shepherd, and Brian Cavanaugh. Emmie and Kevin Burke believe that people who have experienced the trauma of a brain injury and have recovered the skills to live independently and care for others not only understand the needs of the clients but provide them with inspiration. The high ratio of staff to client, roughly one staff member to one client, depending on the house and schedules, accounts for the amount of progress clients have over time achieved.

Hugh Barclay, who has worked at the farm 17 years, is among the staff members who manage clients who live independently. He helps develop jobs for clients and former clients and provides support services to help them stay employed.

In May 1998, Kevin and his sister-in-law Barbara Barron-Rolfe realized the need for an all-women facility, now called Barbara's 1840 House Inc. Located in Rutland, it's the first all- female residential treatment program for women surviving brain injury in Vermont and, perhaps, the only one in the country. Kevin calls it "a Wallingford farmhouse plunked down in the city of Rutland." The handsome, two-story house serves the needs of a clientele that enjoys going to the senior center for bingo and lunch, or to hair or nail appointments, and having the flexibility of a regular bus schedule.

Says Barron-Rolfe, who received the Vermont Governor's Caregiver of the Year Award from Howard Dean in 2001 – one of numerous Governor's Awards given to the organization and its staff – "Here, clients have their own room decorated the way they want," each painted in a color corresponding to the woman's birthstone. Rooms are decorated with photos of kids and grandkids and even great-grandchildren. Barron-Rolfe has taken the whole group of residents to see newborn babies born to residents' children. For example, Louise Beaupre, who was mowed down by a drunk driver while standing in her driveway waiting for a ride to her grandson's basketball game in November 1999, has seen many of her nine grandchildren and one great-grandchild within a day or two of their birth.

Because it's an all-women house, too, decorations are important, especially in winter when Barron-Rolfe hauls out the Christmas Village, decorates Hanukkah and Christmas trees and organizes a neighborhood party complete with horse-drawn rides for the clients and neighborhood kids, with staff aide Diane Esposito dressed as Mrs. Claus.

Says Kevin, "I looked at 12 properties before I chose this one. It was perfect, situated in the southwest neighborhood with all its family traditions. It will be here for years after I'm gone and all the kids who come through here will have met and spent time with these wonderful clients and they will see that a serious injury is not the end of the road."

Among the clients, Stacy, now 34, has been living at Barbara's 1840 House since it opened. She was 14 when she took her mother's car and crashed it, nearly dying as a result. She doesn't speak and must use a wheelchair but her life is full of stimuli, experience and friendship. Until she was 17, she lived with Kevin and his wife Anne, and attended Mill River Union High School. At Barbara's 1840 House, her room, painted in her favorite colors, is decorated with family photos and snapshots taken of her at her senior prom. There she is in her purple gown, smiling radiantly and surrounded by friends.

Somehow along the way, the Burke family members have managed to create their own relationships and families. Kevin and his wife Anne have two children, Sean and Dylan, and four grandchildren. They live in an historic building in Wallingford. Still athletic, Kevin's greatest joy is sharing the out-of-doors with clients, children and grandchildren. And of these outdoor activities, a swim in Chittenden Dam remains on the top of his list. That is, when he's not working. Recent changes in state and federal regulations have placed added demands in record keeping.

In this, he's aided by Jessica Franzoni, a cousin who is the office manager for Lenny Burke's Farm. Kevin describes her as a kind of super-mom, who can talk equally competently to a state or federal bureaucrat and a client. He likes to tell how, when Rev was quite ill, she'd keep one ear listening for the sound of his breathing and the other taking business calls. And then there's Sue Sharp, girl Friday, file keeper and the person who seems to have her finger on the pulse of everything going on at Lenny Burke's Farm and Emmie Burke's household. Of her, Kevin says, "Is there anyone more aptly named?" Sharp is the kind of person who can hear a litany of problems, complications and demands and cut to the chase, devising a solution that satisfies all the demands. Spend a day in this busy office and you'll see that taking care of people with special needs not only generates a lot of paper, but requires a level of organization and bureaucratic skill that seems almost unfathomable. Yet, these three get the job done and still have time to spend with clients. Another Franzoni relative, Robert Franzoni, or as he's called at LBF, Builder Bob, helps the farm stay in compliance by a combination of knowing what is expected in the regulations and being creative in meeting those standards given that all the facilities are old farmhouses, residences or barns.

Kathy was married in Greece. Now single, she lives in Essex, where she cares for her two children, Tommy and Martha. She tries to spend at least one day and evening with her mother and siblings and her children remain close to their grandmother and uncles. She is currently creating a nonprofit organization that will provide stability and activity for people with autism.

Michael Burke has traveled the furthest. After earning an MFA in film production from NYU's Tisch School of the Arts, he became a professor at and subsequently chair of the school's Kanbar Institute of Film and Television in Singapore. He's produced several successful films, including *The Mudge Boy*, which won competitive awards at the Sundance Film Festival and has been featured on Showtime. He lives with his husband, Tai Lam.

Emmie, too, has found a life partner, someone who was there all along. In the years preceding Lenny's injury and for some time after, Lenny's coach Jim Kelley and his former wife Louise were very close to Emmie and Len Burke. The Kelleys had four girls while the Burkes had three boys and a girl, all somewhat the same age. The kids were in sports and other activities together. As happens sometimes when couples marry young, Louise Kelley became unhappy with the relationship and divorced Jim Kelley in the early 1990s.

Emmie and Jim Kelley were cautious with one another but traveled in the same circles and, of course, Kelley loved to visit with Lenny and, unlike Len, was immediately interested in what Emmie was doing at the farm. On the night of New Year's Eve, 1995, Jim was alone while Emmie was having dinner with Lenny at her mother's house in Chittenden, to which she had recently moved. At the spur of a moment, Emmie decided to invite Kelley for dinner. Ever the gentleman, Kelley left that night with a wish to Emmie for a happy new year and a kiss on the cheek, one that gave Emmie an electric charge. That night the barn at Lenny Burke's Farm burned down.

"I like to joke that that spark he gave me burned the whole barn down. I lost a barn but I gained Jim Kelley," Emmie says. "We spent a lot of time together after that. We did Christmas shopping together. We counted on each other. So, since Len had divorced

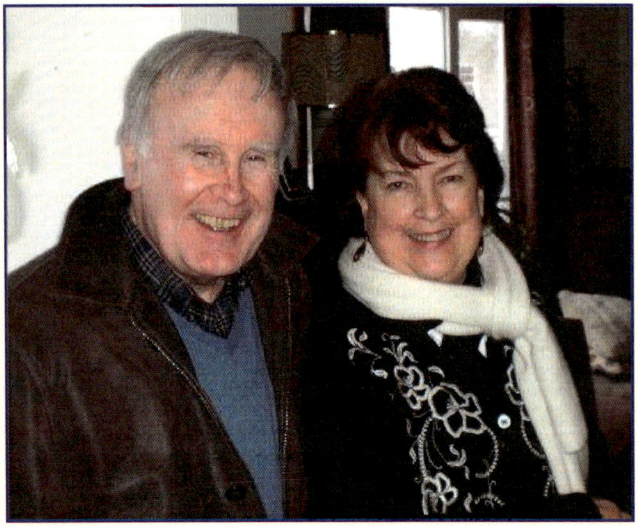

me quite some time before than, there we were. We respected that each other's families were number one. Our relationship just grew. I don't know exactly when things changed and we became special friends but at some point we just decided we would spend more time together," Emmie says. "And that's what we do."

And then there's Lenny, the intrepid youngster whose head injury has brought so many people together and in the deepest way enriched the lives of hundreds. He has an active life in which he golfs when his back allows, visits friends and, with the help of Judy Lowell, his special aide, follows a healthy exercise and rehabilitation schedule. He also likes to go to Friendly's, where all the waitresses vie to wait on him so they can spoil him with an extra scoop of ice cream.

There's someone special in his life too, a woman named Mary Destrempes. Destrempes was a nurse who mentored Lorraine Wargo, a longtime associate of Emmie Burke who was immensely helpful and supportive as the former director of Vermont's Division of Disability and Aging Services. That agency oversaw the Independence Fund grants that allowed Lenny Burke's Farm to come into existence in the first place. Wargo is now executive director of the National Association of State Head Injury Administrators.

Destrempes was 46 when she was struck by an aneurism while attending a conference on educational funding 22 years ago. Now 68, she and Lenny spend two afternoons a week together. Sometimes they paint; sometimes they play cards or watch a movie. The aneurism affected Destrempes' short-term memory but she keeps a little journal in which she writes reminders to herself. The two love the story of what happened when Lenny first asked her to be his girlfriend. Destrempes was excited beyond words. She even joked about being a few years older than her "boyfriend." But the next few times she saw him, she would have forgotten that they had made a commitment to one another and she'd feel the joy all over again. Now that their commitment is safe and happily stored in her long-term memory, she too gets a chuckle out of the story of how she'd forgotten that the two were sweethearts.

Destrempes lives at the Maples, a senior living home in Rutland. She and Lenny are often accompanied by an aide, Maggie Moran, who says this of Lenny: "Lenny has a way of moving into your life – physically, intellectually and emotionally – playfully, lovingly, joyfully, generously, humorously – and always respectfully. He is a wonderful companion."

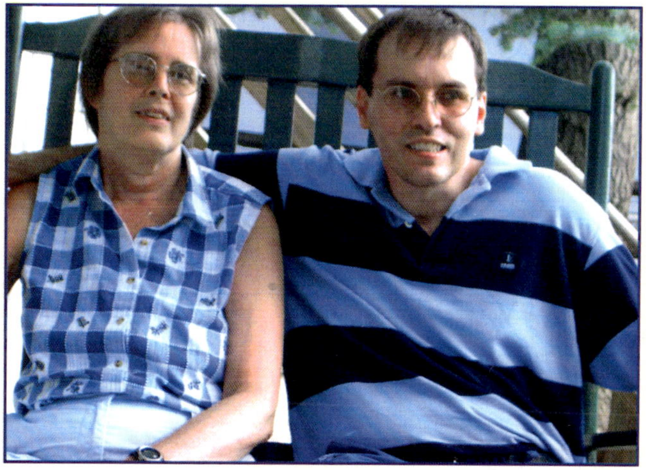

One would think that all this would be enough drama for one family. But another chapter in perseverance and serendipity began to unfold in late 2011 when Len became quite ill and inexplicably was losing a good deal of blood; doctors couldn't figure out what was wrong with him. He'd had many blood transfusions and had been told that he might not live. One day Kevin went to his father's bedside in intensive care to visit with him. Here's how he describes that moment in time: "Two men. Two flawed human beings. No expectations on my part about our roles as father and son, just a willingness to hear him out. Discovery: His heart was broken that night in 1979. He was never able to accept the new Lenny and felt he'd missed 'the party that is Lenny' for 30 years, the party that all of us had been enjoying."

Kevin sat by his father and listened. He thought about how each person has a different version of reality. He gently showed his father a different version of those years, then conceded that nothing could be done about the past but that "We could do something about the future."

As he puts it, "a bridge was built" that allowed Len entry back into the family circle for what was thought to be his last months.

Then, as the Burke siblings began to deal with the impending loss of their father, lightning struck again. Lenny was diagnosed with advanced colon cancer. His life too was in danger. An operation was performed in August 2012, followed by chemotherapy and a long recuperation. Concern ricocheted through Lenny Burke's Farm; Rev had been dead just two years. Now they worried that Lenny, so closely associated with everything the farm stands for, was also fighting for his life.

But then something magical happened. That conversation between Kevin and his father had struck a deep chord. "My father, despite rapidly declining health and strength, decided to use that bridge," Kevin says. As Lenny recuperated from his operation, his father began to spend hours at a time with him in the hospital. Lenny confided to his mother how much the visits meant to him and said something quite typical, the kind of statement that still after all these years amazes those who know him with the depth of his perception and the guileless irony he brings to the most serious situations.

He said, "I'm going to love Dad back into being the best father he ever was."

And that's what happened. Emmie made it clear that Len was welcome to come to her house to visit Lenny upon his release from the hospital. He came every day, sick as he was himself, washed his son and shaved him, then the two would watch sports on the television for hours. For the last seven months of his life, Len was devoted to his son and was instrumental in Lenny's second healing. He died March 18, 2013.

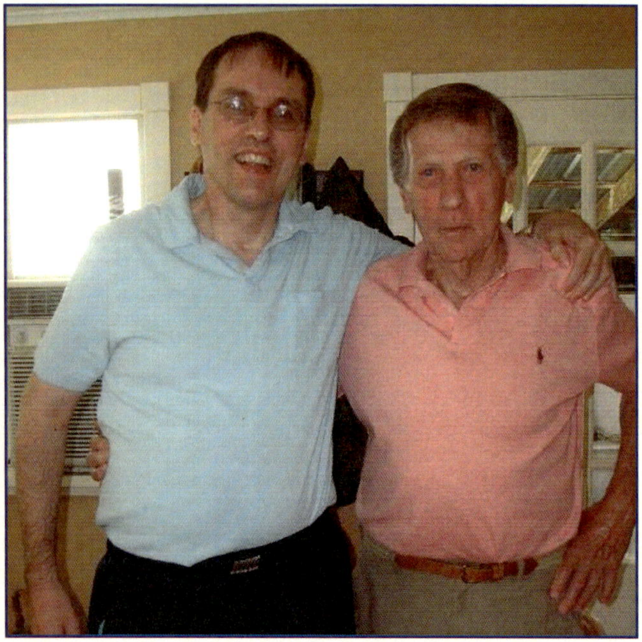

Now, two years out from his surgery, Lenny is cancer free. He's back at the farm a few days a week where he particularly likes Thursday's group when all the clients gather to sing and share stories or the monthly socials that Emmie has long organized, casual gatherings where current and former clients far and wide come together for support, recreation, good food and, most important, a reminder of how far they've come.

At one of those gatherings last summer, former and current clients sat in a circle trading yarns. It soon became apparent that some of the attendees were hearing other clients' stories for the first time. The session went long, almost two hours. But each client listened enthralled as, for example, Bonnie Sawyer spoke of balancing emotional challenges resulting from her brain injury with the success she has had recently composing music. Sawyer, who lives in nearby Clarendon, has never been a formal client at Lenny Burke's Farm but rather is one in a multitude of people who have sustained traumatic brain injuries and come to the monthly support meetings or Thursday group meetings for the comfort of being with others who understand her frustrations.

Martineit, the former computer whiz who lives at the farm, is normally quite shy. But, perhaps responding to the atmosphere of openness in the room, he told the group how frustrated he was when he arrived at Lenny Burke's Farm all those years ago. He told how, after his accident, double vision, near paralysis and memory loss robbed him of so many things that had given him pleasure.

But now, he said, turning to those in the circle, thanks to the services and rehabilitation he's received since coming to the farm, he's working again on the computer and he's found a way to give back to others: once a week, he travels to Genesis Mountainview Center, a nursing home in Rutland, and reads to the residents. And he's talking to his parents about moving closer to them in a more independent setting. His sense of accomplishment filled the room.

Martha Dalton, a woman who works with Dick Bashaw and has been bringing him to the monthly meetings for years, was clearly moved by Martineit's story. "I remember you when you hung your head and said, 'There's nothing you can do for me.' Now, look at you. You've done so well." Then she turned to the whole group and asked, "How many of you here today were told you'd never walk again or something similar about what you couldn't do?"

Hands went up around the room and the stories continued: stories about measuring progress incrementally, yes, but progress nonetheless: new words, new relationships, new challenges.

As the time for the gathering to end neared, everyone turned to Lenny for some parting words about how he was feeling. "You want to know how I'm doing?" he asked. "Look at our clients and you'll see how well I've done. I couldn't be better."

Then he added, "But enough talk. It's cookie time. Let's eat."

"Maybe in the end I see traumatic brain injury like dropping a mirror. At first you see all the broken pieces. Turn it a little to the light and you see all the colors. You look in one piece and you see the whole person, someone unique and special."

—Kathy Chandler, Emma's Place

The Road Continues

No one knows the full implications of one chance encounter or decision. This is true in both the bad way and the good way. We get in the car with our kids to go for a ride; next thing we know, we're in the hospital, or they are, or worse. Or, on the other hand, we make a phone call after doing all we can to help our own child after a horrible injury, talk to a stranger who might help, and make not just a lifelong friend but set in motion a series of events that will lead to discovery after discovery that will help not only one person but thousands others, and each of those encounters and actions will, in and of itself, set in motion a series of other actions.

The College of St. Joseph, where Dr. Ron Savage was working when he was contacted by Emmie Burke for help with her son Lenny, is a small Catholic college located in Rutland, Vermont, far from the centers of scientific research and rehabilitation for something as complex as traumatic brain injury. But Savage was an intense and intelligent man who had an almost obsessive commitment to helping children read better and comprehend what they had read. He'd never worked with someone diagnosed with a brain injury, although later he realized the high possibility that many of his clients may have injured their brains unknowingly. What he learned in helping Lenny changed his life, and thereby others.

In the intervening years, Savage, working with other experts nationally, has lobbied Congress to pass laws to protect people from head injuries and to raise consciousness about the extent and far-ranging impacts of these injuries. As a result of his and so many other people's efforts, sports institutions like the National Football League are being held accountable for the head injuries that athletes can suffer and the behaviors that might result from them.

But as scientists have continued to explore the issue, new conundrums are raised that make us as humans struggle to balance the good that comes of sports and leisure activities with the dangers that we now know are inherently possible. For example, while there has been much attention paid to football, researchers now know that girls soccer ranks second in causing concussions among high school students, followed by wrestling, boys soccer and girls basketball, according to the National Institutes on Health.

But that is only the beginning and we have much to learn. Indeed, if Savage's colleague, Patrick Donohue, is to be believed – and he has substantial research to back up his theory – traumatic brain injury and not cancer, heart disease nor HIV/AIDS is the leading public health crisis of our time. Indeed, Donohue goes so far as to suggest that our prisons are full of people who sustained head injuries when they were children, injuries that were often undiagnosed and therefore untreated.

Savage teamed up with Donohue, the founder of the Sarah Jane Brain Project, several years ago to address the issue of what's called Pediatric Acquired Brain Injury, that is injury to the brain that occurs when children are quite young. Donohue is the founder of the International Academy of Hope in New York City, the first school of its kind designed specifically to serve children who have sustained brain injuries. Savage is the president of the new school.

Begun a year ago with six students, it now has 26. Donohue describes the results of creating and implementing programs specifically designed for individual children's physical, mental, intellectual and emotional needs. Several of the students who arrived unable to walk or talk and whose doctors gave little hope of progress, are now walking, talking and learning. Every child attending the school, he says, has experienced a positive change in both intellectual and physical capability in a very short time.

The need is great for programs like this. Pediatric acquired brain injury is the number-one cause of death and disability for children and young adults in the United States.

It's a subject Donahue is passionate about. He founded the Sarah Jane Donohue Project after his daughter was violently shaken by her baby nurse when she was only five days old, breaking four ribs, both collarbones and causing a pediatric acquired brain injury. Like Emmie Burke, he found that there was no centralized resource for research and rehabilitation about traumatic brain injury in infants nor information for parents such as himself. And, as he began to talk to parents of other children who had sustained pediatric acquired brain injuries, he found that each has had to "invent the wheel" for their child, finding little to rely upon in terms of financial or institutional support.

In time, Donohue came in contact with Savage who invited him to one of the conferences on traumatic brain injury that Savage organizes. Subsequently, Donohue and Savage invited 80 colleagues to New York City to help develop a national "seamless, standardized, evidence-based system of care that is universally accessible for the millions of American families who have a child with a brain injury regardless of where they live."

The statistics they base the need for this program upon are staggering: According to the Centers for Disease Control and Prevention, not only is brain injury the number-one cause of death and disability for American youth and younger adults, but more than 765,000 American youth up to 25 years of age enter an emergency department each year with a new brain injury. Of these, more than 80,000 are hospitalized and over 11,000 die annually.

Says Donohue, "If you compare those numbers to HIV (about 56,000 new cases each year) or autism (about 24,000 new cases each year), you can quickly see how brain injury is a public health crisis."

One hundred and sixty Congressional members have signed onto a bill, HR2600, that would fund these plans and support their implementation for 10 years. It would cost $2.9 billion nationally – Vermont's cost would be $44 million – but the bill has been stalled in the Health, Energy and Commerce Committee because of beltway gridlock.

Donohue says the plan does not require additional funding from Congress after the implementation period and does not create an indefinite new federal program. What it does do, he says, is connect hospitals, schools, treatment centers, medical practitioners, families and their communities together to form a network that will share information and treatment models, updated routinely as research in brain injury and treatment evolves.

Meanwhile, educators in Miami, Dallas, San Francisco, Chicago and a host of other American cities have asked Donohue and Savage to help them create a model school such as the International Academy of Hope and are working to implement the treatment plans on their own, rather than wait for Congress.

Donohue says that the impact on society of traumatic brain injury is much greater than is realized, not just in terms of the children who are diagnosed but also those whose injuries may not be diagnosed or those whose injuries may appear to be minor. He's of the opinion that many young people who commit crimes or otherwise get into difficulty may have had a traumatic brain injury as a child.

As we grow up, decisions require more and more sophisticated and complex reasoning – what's called executive function. Executive functions are controlled by the frontal lobes of the brain. The frontal lobes are connected with many other brain areas and coordinate the activities of these other regions. Indeed, the frontal lobes are often compared to an orchestra's conductor; they communicate with the rest of the brain and help in decision-making.

The major skills that executive function control are: the ability to learn and hold onto information so that it can be used at a later time; the ability to control one's impulses and monitor one's own behavior; and the ability to move within and between tasks and solve problems.

It's not a leap to connect damage to the frontal lobes from a head injury to the kinds of actions that often get young people in trouble – making poor decisions, inability to monitor one's own behavior; failing to learn from past mistakes or to make connections between cause and effect.

Says Donohue, "We know that 765,000 people from birth to 25 years of age go to the emergency room every year as a result of a head injury," and many are deemed to be okay with no follow-up. Indeed, until recently, mild concussions weren't taken as seriously as they are now. He suggests that these injuries manifest themselves in later years when young people need to learn to make their own decisions and are faced with more complex situations and decisions.

"While there has been much attention paid to football, researchers now know that girls soccer ranks second in causing concussions among high school students, followed by wrestling, boys soccer and girls basketball."

–National Institutes on Health

About the Author

Yvonne Daley lives in Rutland, Vermont, where she is the director of the Green Mountain Writers Conference, and San Francisco, where she is a professor of journalism at San Francisco State University. She is the author of four previous books, *An Independent Man* (with Sen. James M. Jeffords); *Vermont Writers: A State of Mind; Octavia Boulevard* and *A Mighty Storm*. She is particularly interested in restorative journalism, the practice of telling true stories with an emphasis on character-driven narrative that not only tells the reader (or viewer) what happened, but looks to the future and the possible lessons to be learned and healing to be sought.

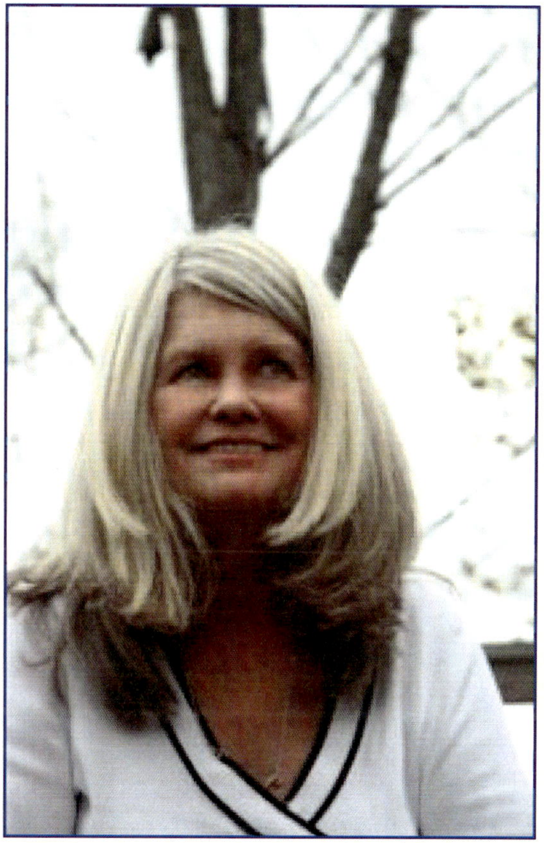

If You Write About Me

By Lenny Burke

If you write about me, don't write that I was a great high school athlete. That's not how I want to be known or remembered. Just say, I was a kind person. I want my story to be about someone who did something kind. That's enough. That's how I want to be remembered. I've had a great life, a happy life. No one could ask for a better life.

Regrets? Sure. Not going to college. Not playing professional sports. I sure wish my golf swing would come back to what it was back then. But I'm alive and surrounded by people who love me. And I love them.

What I miss most is my subconscious. I would cherish nightmares. I miss the sense of smell. But I still like to eat. You can say that about me, the old and the new Lenny both like to eat. Particularly mint chocolate chip ice cream.

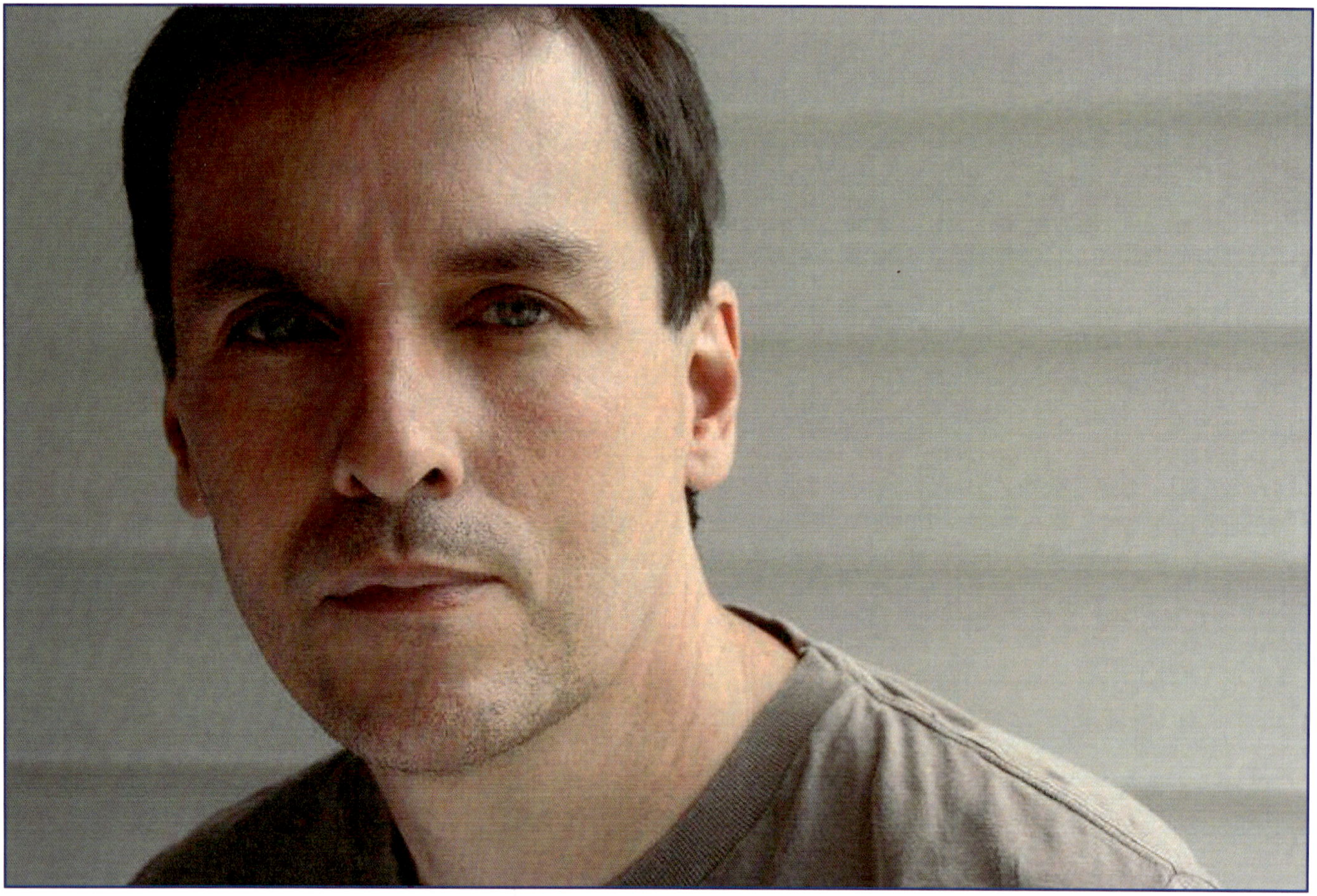

Lenny Burke

CPSIA information can be obtained
at www.ICGtesting.com
Printed in the USA
BVXC01n0151021214
376974BV00004B/6

* 9 7 8 1 6 0 5 7 1 2 3 4 5 *